A Call to Be Whole

The Fundamentals of Health Care Reform

BARBARA J. SOWADA

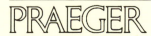

Westport, Connecticut
London

i 0275978850

Library of Congress Cataloging-in-Publication Data

Sowada, Barbara J., 1947–
    A call to be whole : the fundamentals of health care reform / Barbara J. Sowada.
        p.   cm.
Includes bibliographical references and index.
ISBN 0–275–97885–0 (alk. paper)
    1. Health care reform—United States. I. Title.
RA395.A3S763   2003
362.1′0425—dc21   2002044951

British Library Cataloguing in Publication Data is available.

Library of Congress Catalog Card Number: 2002044951
ISBN: 0–275–97885–0

First published in 2003

Praeger Publishers, 88 Post Road West, Westport, CT 06881
An imprint of Greenwood Publishing Group, Inc.
www.praeger.com

Printed in the United States of America

The paper used in this book complies with the
Permanent Paper Standard issued by the National
Information Standards Organization (Z39.48–1984).

10 9 8 7 6 5 4 3 2 1

In memory of Patty Ann Riley

Contents

Illustrations

TABLES

Acknowledgments

It's a pleasure to thank the persons whose help and support made this book possible. I am particularly grateful to two special people whose encouragement focused and sustained me during the seven years I spent refining my thinking and writing: Bernadette Prinster, M.S., Director, Community End of Life Care Network Project, Santa Fe, NM; and Mitch Saunders, President, Action Learning Partners, Felton, Calif.

I also wish to thank Sister Lynn Casey of the Sisters of Charity of Leavenworth and former CEO of St. Mary's Hospital & Medical Center, the participants of the Grand Junction Dialogue Project, and the project's facilitators—William N. Isaacs, Mitch Saunders, Barbara Coffman, John Gray, and their support staff.

For the grass root examples, I am grateful to CeCe Huffnagle, R.N., N.P., Woman's Health and Menopause Center, Denver, Colo.; Beth Branthaver, Manager, Chronic Conditions Management Program, Kaiser Permanente of Northern California; John Huddler, Editor, Burlington Record, Burlington, Colo.; James Glaser, Director, Center for Healthcare Reform, St. Joseph Health System, Orange, Calif., a ministry of the Sisters of St. Joseph of Orange; and Janet Cameron, Executive Director, Marillac Clinic, Grand Junction, Colo., a ministry of the Sisters of Charity of Leavenworth; and Sylvia McSkimming, Executive Director, Supportive Care of the Dying. To the many people whose personal experience or composite experiences were used to illustrate the strengths and weaknesses of the current health care system, I also owe a debt of gratitude.

Gratitude is due as well to Foy Ritchie, President, Rocky Mountain Pastoral Care and Training Associates, for the information regarding reconcil-

iation. I am also grateful to those who read parts of the draft of the manu-
script: Julie Barak, Donna Crouch, Pam Curlee, Katherine Ellis, Linda
Evans, Carol Farina, Michelle Hansen, William N. Isaacs, Ann Leadbetter,
Bernadette Prinster, Jane Quimby, Mitch Saunders, June Simonton, Karen
Speerstra, Tom Tompkins, and John Zeigel.

Thanks, too, to graphic artist Laura Bradley; the team at Impressions
Book and Journal Services, Inc.; and Halley Gatenby, copyeditor. Even
with the help of those mentioned, this book wouldn't have happened
without the support of my husband, Robert Sowada. Finally, any mistakes
are solely mine.

Introduction

Beware what you set your heart upon. For it surely shall be yours.
Ralph Waldo Emerson

Today, it is common for politicians and pundits to call for public dialogue to resolve any one of health care's numerous intractable problems or its myriad of moral dilemmas. Whenever I hear the call for public dialogue, a frisson of alternating currents—anxiety and hopefulness—runs up my spine. Having participated in a two-year dialogue regarding health care reform, I am convinced that public dialogue holds the solution to health care's problems. The conviction is paradoxical: Dialogue challenges us to move beyond the existing limits of our relationships and tests our willingness to care for one another.

In 1992, health care reform was a presidential campaign issue. Campaign watchwords included *universal health care* and *quality at an affordable price*. For those of us working in health care, it was as though a terrible, fire-breathing dragon were rumbling our way. There wasn't anyone inside health care who didn't sense the high-stakes implications of health care reform. On the outside, the public watched, hoping that health care reform would include some alternative care, nursing home coverage for their elderly parents, and health insurance for the entire family, all at an affordable price. When the smoke cleared, however, health care reform had defaulted to politically correct economic issues, much to the public's sorrow.

Dialogue was finding its way into the U.S. vocabulary, and its effectiveness for facilitating social change was at the exploratory stage. That year, I was one of three women who catalyzed our local community to participate in a research project using dialogue for health care reform. The experiment, known locally as the Grand Junction Dialogue Project, was an action research initiative sponsored by the Organizational Learning Center at the Massachusetts Institute of Technology. The researchers' purpose was to develop practical knowledge regarding dialogue as a vehicle for social change. The community's goal was to find its own responses to health care reform initiatives that were then sweeping the health care landscape.

The Dialogue Project met in Grand Junction, Colorado, from January through May 1993 and from January through October 1994. The thirty-eight-member local group included physicians, nurses, and executives from the five local hospitals, the local Health Maintenance Organization (HMO) and the county health department. A state legislator, several business and community leaders, and consumers further diversified the locals. Each represented institution had independent strategies and philosophies for providing health care and for decades had operated in a state of entrenched competition. The CEOs of two competing hospitals had never been inside each other's facility. The strong difference in education, responsibilities, privileges, and expectations among the providers—doctors, nurses, allied health practitioners, and administrators—further complicated the competitive atmosphere. That this diverse, competitive group came together was itself a miracle.

The Dialogue Project was a bold and courageous move, but it was only a fragile beginning. At its end, I was left with more questions than answers. Were health care's problems really so intractable? Why were bright people with good intentions unable to collaborate? What did project members miss or overlook? Bernadette Prinster, one of the project's catalysts, and I explored these questions for the next two years, an inquiry encouraged by Mitch Saunders, one of the researchers of the project.

As the information accrued, Bernadette and I realized that the thirty-eight of us presumed we were talking about the same health care system, but in fact we were not. The group, dominated by providers, took the definition of health for granted. Largely ignoring the different definitions of health that are in play today meant that members of the group didn't clearly see what they were attempting to reform.

Multiple definitions of health means there is no one coherent picture of health care. Instead, there are many images of health care and many more ideas about the cause, prevention, and cure of disease. Some images are nascent and emerging, and others, such as Norman Rockwell's image of a kindly, fatherlike physician, are outmoded and receding. In short, given health care's complexities and the many images of health care, reform is bound to fail. It cannot succeed until we begin to understand the deeper issues and see clearly what is actually being reformed.

Looking back, the project's problem resided in our own thinking, steeped in Newtonian physics and Cartesian thought. Our conversations tacitly recapitulated three beliefs that society largely takes for granted: Health care is an independent entity, money and morals are separate issues, and facts are more truthful than feelings. From my present vantage point, I see that we were not aware of our own ignorance regarding multiple definitions of health and care. It never occurred to us to question the schizophrenic beliefs inherent in the modern health care system. Moreover, we were very much afraid of loss of control and more attentive to the national political scene than we cared to admit to one another.

We were simply too enmeshed in the health care system to see it clearly. Although we understood that health care, like all social systems, is generated from thought, we couldn't see that the thought that created health care is the source of its problems. We took what we thought of as given and about as close to the truth as one could come. Had we only realized that our competitive local relationships actually came from the same source of thinking that continues to foster the national piecemeal attempts at reform, the project might well have ended altogether differently.

This book is the result of my inquiry into the thought that generates the modern health care system. In order to reveal the deeper issues and clearly show the complex interrelationships that inform the structure and function of health care, in this book I inquire into four age-old questions that shape all health care systems:

1. What is health?
2. What is care?
3. How much is enough?
4. Who is responsible?

The inquiry has four purposes. The first is to help the reader see how the answers to the four questions define the structure and function of health care. The second, because health care is a part of a nested hierarchy of systems—self, health care, market economy, and worldview—is to show the effect of the other systems on the modern configuration of health care and to explain why health care cannot be re-formed without evoking changes in the other systems. The third is to illuminate the deeper issues underlying today's access, cost, and quality problems and to show that these problems are interrelated and arise from outmoded organizing concepts, unquestioned assumptions, and a long trail of inconsistent and contradictory answers to the four questions. The fourth purpose is to acquaint readers with both the personal and the societal challenges of finding coherent answers to the four questions and to describe some of the budding experimental solutions that challenge traditional conventions and common wisdom.

This book invites readers to explore their own beliefs. Readers working their way through the inquiry are apt to discover that their answers, which over time have helped maintain the current system, are seldom free of social conditioning. Many will be surprised at how frequently their answers to one question contradict their answers to one or more of the other questions. Others will be dismayed that there are no magic bullets and no sound-byte answers to painful issues regarding the purpose of health care or to the very real limits of resources and of life itself. More than anything, readers must ask themselves the deepest question they can ask: What does it mean to care for other human beings?

ORGANIZATION

This book is divided into three broad sections. Like a magnetic resonance image (MRI), the chapters are arranged layer by layer until the dynamic, complex, undisassociable configuration of health care is exposed. The recursive design is intentional: Human beings and their systems are mutually enfolded. Ineluctably, health care's structure and function reflect the values and beliefs imprinted on its designers' minds. To change health care is to change our minds.

The first section presents an overview of health care and of systems. Chapter 1 explains why health care is a trillion-dollar industry and why the market can neither control health care costs nor reform the health care system. Chapter 2 explains health care's theoretical foundation and describes why the health care crisis is a call to heal what thought has fractured. The second section reveals the confusion. Chapters 3, 4, 5, and 6 inquire into the four age-old questions that shape all health care systems and show the extent to which economic, scientific, and philosophic forces shape our answers. At the end of each of these four chapters is a set of questions designed to expand readers' awareness of their own beliefs regarding the meaning and purpose of health care. The third section explores reconciling relationships. Chapter 7 claims that many of the solutions to health care reform are known and that the resistance to implementing those solutions is due to fears of loss. Chapter 8, which returns the readers to themselves, is a reminder that health care can never be better than the relationships of those involved and that dialogue can transcend reductionistic thought, reconciling seemingly disparate parts into a more coherent whole. Finally, Chapter 9 looks forward to new beginnings and reminds us that by healing health care we also heal ourselves.

Before we begin our process of unpacking health care, let me close this introduction with several disclaimers. First, although this book stands on the shoulders of the Grand Junction Dialogue Project, this book is not about the Grand Junction Dialogue Project. The project has been described elsewhere. Second, this book is not intended to be a comprehensive analysis or a final solution, but an inquiry into the complex relationships among human beings and their systems. Intended as a careful sorting out, or an unpacking of the thought that generates the structure and function of the modern health care system, it is an attempt to bring some order and understanding into the morass of contentious and confusing economic and moral issues now perturbing health care's stability. Third, inquiry, which has the potential for taking us to new levels of understanding, is about asking questions and moving us ever deeper into thought. Thus readers should consider the threads of information I have surfaced as starting points for their own investigation into the challenges of and possibilities for health care reform. Finally, I don't expect everyone to share my beliefs, though they are obvious: that life and resources are limited, that we can see what the heart can hold, and that what we choose for our neighbor we ultimately choose for ourselves. Finally, by healing the health care system we become more fully human.

CHAPTER 1

Heartburn

First do no harm.

—Hippocratic Oath

"What's wrong with health care?" Chances are, most Americans would say health care costs too much, that they are spending more and getting less. Health care is expensive and gets ever more expensive. Costs have risen from 5.3 percent of the gross domestic product (GDP) in 1960 to roughly 14 percent in 2000. Health care is now a $1.3 trillion industry, consuming about one-sixth of the U.S. economy. Of the $1.3 trillion, about 45 percent comes from taxes, 34 percent from insurance premiums, and 15 percent directly from patients' pockets. Health care costs the average household $8,000 annually, according to C. E. Steuerle of the Urban Institute.[1]

Americans have reason to worry that health care will be priced out of reach. All too often, those with health insurance lose their coverage through no fault of their own, becoming part of the 20 percent, or 43 million, without health insurance—a number that has grown by a million persons annually since the early 1980s. The elderly worry about the price of prescription drugs; low wage earners can't afford health insurance coverage for their children; some people with insurance can't afford the co-payments and deductibles. Still others are forced into bankruptcy by uncovered medical bills. Disastrous medical bills account for about 40 percent of the bankruptcies filed in 1999.[2]

Access and quality are also concerns. The media is full of stories about disappearing services and denied benefits. It seems that most of the public knows someone personally who was turned away by a doctor, a hospital, or an insurance company. The effects range from petty annoyance to moral outrage. Having to petition for prior approval or having a health plan dictate the physicians and hospitals one can go to is irritating, but it's outrageous that many working people do not have health care benefits and that many elderly have to choose between buying prescription drugs and paying their heating bill.

Because health care is something we may not be able to live without, each of us has a personal interest in health care reform. Chances are, we have an opinion about why health care costs so much and what should be done to fix it. Some blame waste, claiming that 30–50 percent of health care costs are due to unnecessary tests and procedures, duplication of services, and an oversupply of physicians. Some blame it on greed, noting the high incomes of physicians, the hefty profit margins of insurance companies and hospitals, and price-gouging by purveyors of pharmaceuticals and medical goods. Some point to medical fraud and litigious patients. Still others blame the high costs on extravagant overhead, comparing Canada's 10 percent to the United States' 21 percent overhead costs. Yet very few of us would claim we ourselves contribute to health care's soaring costs.

IS HEALTH CARE A RIGHT OR A PRIVILEGE?

Health care, like education, is part of the infrastructure of industrialized societies. Historically, the moral role industrial societies have ascribed to health care falls between two extremes. At one end is the notion that health care is a consumer good, like cars and clothing, whose financing is the responsibility of individual consumers. At the other end, health care is considered a social good that is collectively financed and available to all who need it. Whereas European countries long ago decided that health care is a social good, the United States has never reached political consensus. Instead, health care here waffles between these two roles depending upon the political climate of the time.[3]

European countries, whose economies are similar to ours, have had some form of national insurance since the late 1800s. Years ago, Europeans tied health insurance to a general social insurance program that not only underwrites medical care but also protects laborers against the loss of income due to sickness and disability, industrial accidents, old age, and unemployment. In contrast, Americans have not yet agreed whether health care is a right or a privilege. Even though roughly half of health care costs are paid for by a combination of federal, state, and local taxes, the United States is the only industrialized country, except for South Africa, whose government doesn't guarantee the right to health care by providing universal health benefits to all its citizens.

Despite multiple attempts throughout the twentieth century, the United States has never enacted any form of universal health benefits. Presidents Woodrow Wilson, Harry Truman, John Kennedy, and Jimmy Carter advocated universal and comprehensive national health insurance. These plans, like the Bill Clinton plan, fell prey to the lobbying efforts of the American Medical Association (AMA) and other special interest groups who play on the public's fear of socialized medicine. Instead of having a uniform system like the Europeans, the United States has a crazy quilt of entrepreneurial practices, stitched together by a wide range of often conflicting governmental policies.

HEALTH CARE AS AN ECONOMIC GAME

Since the 1930s, considerable effort has been spent on making health care affordable to the general public. Despite seventy years of effort, costs continue to rise. Americans have the most costly health care system in the world, yet it ranks thirty-seventh in keeping people healthy, according to World Health Organization data from 2000.[4]

The model that best describes the current health care system is that of a continuous economic circular game—much like the children's game of musical chairs—with six groups of players, or stakeholders: patients, providers, payers, purchasers, purveyors of medical goods and pharmaceuticals, and politicians. *Payers* is shorthand for third-party payers, or the insurance component of health care, and *purchasers* is jargon for businesses, the major purchasers of health insurance for non-elderly people. Politicians, especially representatives of the federal government, are more powerful than the other stakeholders because they can enact legislation that affects the others. Also, the government wields tremendous purchasing power, funding Medicare and Medicaid and underwriting major portions of graduate medical education and capital construction costs.

The purpose of the game is not health, but economic growth, and the score is kept in dollars. Basically, each group of players wants to minimize its costs, or—to put it another way—to maximize its profits. Because the players are circularly linked, the action of one group automatically either adds to or subtracts from the profits of one or more of the other players (see Figure 1.1).

The game forms an observable pattern. The purchaser (usually an employer or the government) buys health insurance; the patients are treated by providers (typically, physicians and hospitals); the payer (the insurance carrier) pays the providers a negotiated amount; and the patient pays the co-payments, deductibles, and coinsurance costs. As with all well-entrenched patterns, this process is repeated over and over in regular and predictable ways.

THE ADVENT OF PRIVATE HEALTH INSURANCE

Prior to the advent of insurance, health care was mostly supplied by solo practitioners charging whatever the market would bear. The wealthy

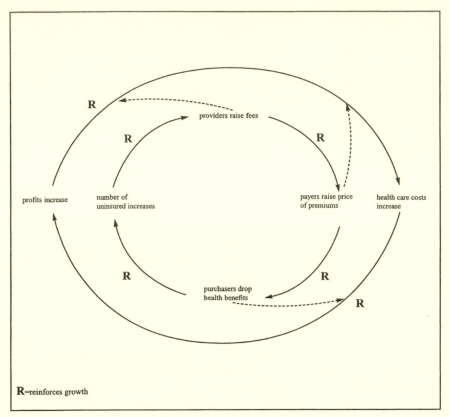

Figure 1.1 Quest to Maximize Profits

paid more, the less wealthy paid less, and the poor—if they received care—were given care through charity.

The Great Depression forced many people to forgo health care; many of those who sought care were often unable to pay. For most people, the little money they had in their pockets went to food, rent, and other necessities. Doctors and hospitals typically waited months to be paid or were not paid at all. The precipitously rising payment deficits threatened hospital viability. By 1932, the American Hospital Association recognized that hospital insurance was the practical solution to the problem.

The original U.S. model for health insurance was Blue Cross and Blue Shield. Blue Cross was started during the depression in Texas by Baylor Hospital, which provided schoolteachers with up to twenty-one days of hospital care for the prepayment of six dollars per month. The plan relieved teachers of the burden of hospital bills, and it gave Baylor a guaranteed revenue stream. Despite fierce opposition from the American

Medical Association (AMA), hospitals found the plan so valuable that by the late 1930s, Blue Cross plans were in every state, insuring millions of people.

An adamant proponent of solo practitioners and fee-for-service reimbursement, the AMA opposed any form of health insurance, for the AMA feared insurance would lead to national health insurance and the subsequent loss of physician autonomy. Finally, in 1942, as a reaction against the popular, consumer-managed health insurance cooperatives and as a preferable alternative to national health insurance, the AMA approved of insurance *if* doctors controlled the plan, opening the way for Blue Shield.

To preserve their status as independent entrepreneurs, physicians wanted control and insisted that Blue Shield be fee-for-service, indemnity plans. *Fee-for-service* means providers set their own fees, unconstrained by an externally imposed fee schedule. *Indemnity* means that the provider bills the patient, not the insurance company, and the insurer reimburses the patient, although not necessarily the full amount. The design was a windfall to physicians. Blue Cross guaranteed physicians payment for the care of low-income patients, though not necessarily the full amount; and paying the full amount—patients with higher incomes—would still pay more.

Blue Cross and Blue Shield formed an ensemble that protected each other's interests. Their financial arrangements assured physician control over health care, for even if other practitioners (such as midwives or naturopathic doctors) could circumvent licensing laws, Blue Shield or other insurers usually did not cover their services. In return, doctors and hospitals boycotted plans they did not control or that imposed a predetermined fee schedule. This gave the Blues a competitive advantage in the nascent health insurance marketplace.

By World War II, one of five Americans was insured against hospital costs, with Blue Cross garnering three-fourths of the market share. Protection against other kinds of medical expense, such as drugs and physician office visits, was not common until after the war.

TYING HEALTH INSURANCE TO EMPLOYMENT

The Taft-Hartley Act

The Taft-Hartley Act of 1947 was a political compromise to President Truman's plan for universal and comprehensive national health insurance. Truman wanted a national program to assure all Americans access to adequate medical care and protection from the economic hazards of sickness. Fearing that a national program would diminish its monopolistic control and erode its authority in the medical marketplace, the AMA vehemently opposed Truman's plan as "socialized medicine."[5]

Instead of a plan to include all Americans, a political compromise made health benefits a part of collective bargaining. Believing that adding health benefits would boost union membership, union leaders supported the compromise. Workers found the agreement attractive since health benefits were nontaxable income and the unions usually bargained for a generous benefits package. By the end of 1954, about 60 percent of the population had some type of hospital insurance, 50 percent had some type of surgical insurance, and about 25 percent had medical insurance (though often only for in-hospital services).[6] Employer-based coverage peaked in 1987, with roughly 70 percent of the non-elderly population receiving health insurance as an employment benefit. By 2000, about 61 percent of the non-elderly had health insurance through their employment.[7]

Employee Retirement Income Security Act

In 1974, employers entered the health insurance arena with the passage of the Employee Retirement Income Security Act (ERISA), a federal law governing employee benefits plans. Written to protect employee pension plans, this law also permits employers to be *self-insured*, or to act as their own health insurance carrier.

Unlike the Blues or commercial carriers, such as Prudential, which are subject to state insurance regulation, self-insured employers are subject to federal ERISA provisions. This disparity contributes to the high cost of health care. The number of state-mandated health insurance benefit laws has risen from 48 in 1970 to more than 1,000 in 1991, and the variety of special interests benefits range from heart transplants in Georgia, to hairpieces in Minnesota, to marriage counseling in California and sperm banks in Massachusetts. Most states have also enacted laws regarding the coverage of HIV treatment, substance abuse, and mental health issues. Because ERISA exempts self-insured businesses from state-mandated benefits, the cost of mandated benefits falls on small firms and purchasers of individual policies who, not large enough to be self-insured, must rely on commercial insurance.[8]

While state regulations require carriers to provide a minimum standard of benefits, ERISA does not mandate either the size or the scope of benefits packages. ERISA also allows employers to reduce health benefits without warning to employees and prohibits employees from suing self-insured employers for malpractice. Finally, ERISA prohibits states from requiring employers to offer benefits to their employees. Because of ERISA, employers have no legal obligation to provide health benefits to their workers. Instead, the provision of health benefits depends upon the company's philosophy, whether it can afford the premiums, and its need to attract highly skilled workers.

EXPENSIVE CONSEQUENCES

The Taft-Hartley Act was a mixed blessing, creating as many economic problems as it solved. Although the majority of Americans had health insurance benefits for the first time, the nonproductive were excluded. Coverage for children, the unemployed, and the poor remains a persistent and intractable problem, as does coverage for nonunionized workers.

Even though health benefits are largely tied to employment, employment is not necessarily tied to health benefits. Eighty-six percent of the uninsured work, albeit at the low end of the wage scale; 54 percent have full-time jobs, and 32 percent work part-time. The problem is, they work at jobs where employers don't—or can't afford to—offer health benefits, or if benefits are offered, the employees can't afford their share of the costs or can't afford to insure their families. In contrast, only 11 percent of adults who earn $35,000 to $59,999 and 3 percent earning $60,000 or more are uninsured.[9]

About 60 percent of American workers have health insurance today, but these benefits are not guaranteed. Despite the 1996 Kennedy Kassenbaum legislation, which theoretically makes health care benefits portable, insurers are free to charge whatever they want. Since a replacement policy can cost as much as $15,000 a year, losing one's job, changing jobs, retiring, or even having an extended illness often translates into lost benefits.

Health insurance expanded the health care market and inflated prices, benefiting providers and payers. Hospital care doubled in price during the 1950s, and physicians' incomes rose 5.9 percent per year, compared to the consumer price index annual increase of 2.8 percent. Moreover, the rapid growth of employer-sponsored health insurance was immediately followed by an equally rapid rise in the number of commercial health insurance carriers. By 1990, the United States had approximately 1,500 carriers, each with its own costly administrative, overhead, and marketing costs.

To compete with the well-entrenched Blues, who based premiums on a *community rating* (that is, everyone in the group pays the same premium), the commercial insurers entered the market by offering lower rates to younger, healthier groups. Under a risk-stratifying system known as *experience rating*, patients are categorized according to age, sex, race, health status, and other probabilities of risk. Those with the highest risk pay the highest premium rates. By the 1970s, most insurers were using experience rating.

Left with growing numbers of more expensive patients, the Blues were forced to continuously raise their rates. By pricing their rates just below the Blues' rising rates, the commercials gradually pulled up the overall cost of premiums.

The insurance industry–led competitive shift away from community rating to experience rating was a pivotal event in the history of health care financing. With community rating, risks are pooled and costs are shared with the understanding that "I don't need health care today, but I might tomorrow." In contrast, with experience rating, premiums are not based on the cost of caring for people over their life span but are calculated according to quarterly corporate profits. Because each risk classification is expected to make a profit, experience rating eventually pushes the high risk patients out of the market.

MEDICARE AND MEDICAID

As part of President Lyndon Johnson's Great Society, Medicare and Medicaid were enacted to protect the elderly, the disabled, and the poor from the economic hazards of sickness. Conceptually, Medicare and Medicaid are radically different programs.

Originally, Medicare beneficiaries included the elderly and people who have been disabled for more than twenty-four months. Later, Medicare included people on kidney dialysis and the terminally ill. Medicare has a standardized benefits package. Briefly, Part A, which is mandatory, includes hospitalization, out-patient services, skilled nursing facilities, and hospice care. Part B, which is optional for a monthly fee, pays a portion of physician fees and some physician-prescribed therapies, such as physical therapy or cardiac rehabilitation therapy. Drugs, dental care, and eyeglasses are not covered.

Medicare was designed for acute care, not for catastrophic or chronic sicknesses. It was also designed to include deductibles and co-payments, both of which have greatly increased over time. By the mid-1990s, Medicare covered about 45 percent of the health care costs incurred by those over age sixty-five. To cover the remaining 55 percent, about 80 percent of the elderly purchase a supplementary insurance policy.

Medicaid, in contrast, is built on the public assistance model and is funded by general taxes. Medicaid is a joint federal-state program with the federal government paying about half the costs—more for the poorer states and less for the wealthier ones. Adding to the overall chaos in the system, the fifty states have made very different decisions about how many services they will cover and who is eligible. Briefly, the states' enrollment criteria are so strict that fewer than half of residents whose incomes are below the poverty line qualify. Unlike Medicare, Medicaid does not include co-payments and deductibles. Because its payments are set so low, not all physicians will care for Medicaid patients.

Contrary to popular opinion, the bulk of Medicaid does not go to unwed mothers. Data from the Urban Institute shows that about 30 percent of Medicaid monies pay for nursing home care for baby boomers' elderly parents, who represent about 11 percent of its beneficiaries. About 38 percent pays for the care of the disabled. Another 25 percent pays for the care of low-income children from single-parent families who represent 50 percent of the Medicaid population, and 12 percent of Medicaid dollars goes to non-disabled adults.[10]

For the first time, many poor and elderly people had access to health care. In 1963, 19 percent of Americans living beneath the poverty level had never been examined by a physician. By 1970, this number had dropped to 8 percent. The most noticeable benefit was the 33 percent drop in the infant mortality rate among the poor between 1965 and 1975.[11]

Like the earlier attempts at national health care legislation, Medicare/ Medicaid faced stiff political opposition from physicians and other special interest groups. The political rhetoric made it perfectly clear that the legislation was *not* to establish the right to health care. Instead, as the conceptual differences between Medicare and Medicaid reflect, the legislation conformed to America's entrepreneurial, piecemeal, and class-oriented approach to health care. Class sentiment is apparent in the public's attitude toward each program.[12] The attitude toward Medicare is, "I am entitled, I paid for it." In contrast, "I've already paid once for me, so why should I have to pay for you as well?" is the general sentiment of the middle class toward Medicaid recipients.

To gain physician and hospital support, legislators made three significant concessions. First, in keeping with the Blue Shield and Blue Cross model, Medicare paid physicians and hospitals separately. Both types of providers were guaranteed they would continue to receive the traditional fee-for-service reimbursement, or be paid on a *cost plus* basis. That is, the government would not impose a fixed fee schedule but instead would pay the provider's costs plus a reasonable profit. Second, hospitals extracted an additional reimbursement for capital equipment, which reinforced the acquisition of new technology and greatly strengthened the financial position of the hospital industry. Third, the law provided for fiscal intermediaries. Placing the administration of Medicare and Medicaid in the hands of the private insurance sector killed two birds with one stone. The concession actively avoided the doctors' and the hospitals' fears of government encroachment on medical authority, and it increased revenues within the insurance sector because the intermediaries were paid for reimbursements, consulting, and auditing services.

The concessions reinforced the growth of the insurance industry, maintained physicians' control over health care, and reinforced health care's entrepreneurial underpinnings. Intended to protect the poor and the elderly from the economic fears of sickness, government spending instead launched the lucrative medical-industrial complex.

FEE-FOR-SERVICE REINFORCES MARKET
EXPANSION

Unlike other markets, in which consumer demand and ability to pay largely determine market growth, health care is *not* controlled by consumers. This condition is reinforced by health care's structure. On one hand, consumers, lacking scientific expertise, tend to turn over every health-related decision to their doctors. On the other, insurers pay by units of care, and licensing laws give physicians control over the demand. By law, patients cannot order their own CT scans or prescribe antibiotics for their children.

The availability of seemingly unlimited monies with almost no cost controls or regulation of medical practice is a potent incentive to raise prices, provide more services, and add new services, especially when combined with capital reimbursement incentives. Consequently, the United States has more nursing homes, hospital beds, diagnostic laboratories, dialysis centers, and rehabilitation centers than any other nation. In fact, Boston, like most big cities, has about twice as many hospital beds as it needs; there are more MRIs in the city of Denver than in all of Canada; and the United States has four times as many mammography machines as would be needed if every woman had a mammogram twice a year.

Moreover, subsidizing both the supply of and demand for technology reinforces health care's dependence on technology (see Figure 1.2). On one hand, capital reimbursement incentives reinforce the acquisition of technology. On the other, the use of the newest technology tends to generate greater revenues for physicians because newer technology generally has higher reimbursement rates.

In other industries, an increase in supply usually drives down costs. In health care, an increase in supply drives costs up. With a surplus of physicians, hospital beds, and diagnostic services, the worried well and patients with self-limiting conditions have ready access to medical care, artificially inflating demand. Excess capacity not only increases volume but also increases overall costs. Physician and hospital charges are generally higher in areas where there is excess capacity, patients are hospitalized more frequently, and the excess care is mostly provided by specialists, who tend to order more expensive tests and procedures than do general practitioners.

Overutilization of services, which is the provision of unnecessary or futile care, is a significant issue. Since the early 1970s, numerous studies have shown wide variations by geographical area in the use of medical services that have no correlation with clinical criteria. That hysterectomies are twice as prevalent in some regions of the country, that more babies are delivered by cesarean section than need to be, that men living in affluent communities are more likely to have coronary artery bypass surgery than

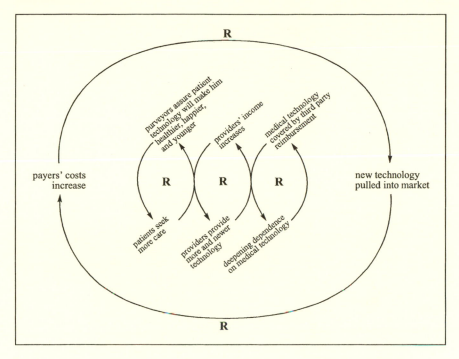

Figure 1.2 Technology and Fee-for-Service Reimbursement Reinforce Each Other's Growth

their less-affluent neighbors are explained more by the way providers are reimbursed than by medical need. Some estimate that the combination of too many specialists, excess capacity, and overutilization accounts for up to 30 percent of total health care expenditures.

Fee-for-service reimbursement coupled with large amounts of Medicare monies and capital reimbursement incentives is a potent formula for economic growth. Patients do not have to be responsible consumers but turn over their care to their doctor, trusting that he or she will provide them with every available intervention with the slightest potential benefit. Providers are *not* paid by outcome, or by whether the patient's health has improved, but are paid by unit of service.

In this economic game, the provider's costs—plus a profit margin—are passed to the payer. The payer tacks on its profit margin and passes its costs to the purchaser: the employer or the government. The circle is completed as employers tack on their insurance costs to the price tags of their products, and the government raises taxes. Taxpayers pick up about half of U.S. health care costs. As long as each party was willing to absorb the costs for the next round of market expansion, all seemed well.

PIECEMEAL ECONOMIC REFORM

By the early 1970s, businesses were no longer willing to absorb the high costs of health care into their production costs. Business was facing the lowest level of corporate profits since World War II, but health care was booming. Health insurance and fee-for-service reimbursement had made health care nearly recession proof.

Sympathetic to businesses' interests, and as the largest purchaser of health care, the federal government was also interested in reducing its costs. Besides widespread concerns over costs and inefficiencies, critics also cited growing issues about patients' rights and uneven access to care. And, for the first time, health care was criticized for its ineffectiveness at keeping people healthy.

There was again talk of national health insurance. Instead, policy analysts proposed that costs could be contained by making health care responsive to the forces of the marketplace. The solution, to make health care "function like a business," and health maintenance organizations (HMOs) were proposed as the corporate solution. The HMO legislation signed by President Richard Nixon pursued market mechanisms: investment incentives, deregulation, and competition. These incentives were expanded and intensified during the Ronald Reagan–George H. W. Bush years. In addition, Medicare/Medicaid's fee-for-service reimbursement was replaced with *prospective reimbursement,* a pre-established rate schedule.

These policy changes set off a cascade of profit-protecting adjustment within the purchaser, payer, and provider sectors. In the twenty years it would take for HMOs to dominate the marketplace, the complementary legislation of the Nixon and Reagan administrations reconfigured health care into a corporate enterprise.

The Reagan administration replaced Medicare/Medicaid's fee-for-service reimbursement with prospective reimbursement, which the commercial insurance companies quickly adopted. Known as *DRGs,* Diagnostic Related Groups are a pre-established reimbursement schedule based on the severity of the condition. For instance, gall bladder surgery paid less than the more complicated coronary bypass surgery. To encourage providers to be efficient, rates were fixed, regardless of the type or amount of services used.

Medicaid made access more difficult. Since Medicaid legislation prohibited co-payments and deductibles, patient-driven demand was controlled by reducing Medicaid enrollment through more stringent eligibility requirements. On the physician side of the equation, Medicaid's deeply discounted fee schedule is so low that many providers will not care for Medicaid patients.

Prospective reimbursement caused profit-protecting adjustments within the provider sector. Doctors and hospitals soon learned to capitalize on the new regulations. To maximize their revenue, they billed at the highest reasonably feasible DRG code, and they *unbundled* services—reporting as multiple procedures what used to be coded as one procedure. Also, doctors began charging for such things as phone calls, follow-up visits, and other things that previously were included as part of a procedure.

Until 1995, DRGs applied only to inpatient care. Because outpatient services continued to be paid for by fee-for-service reimbursement, providers quickly shifted as much care as possible to outpatient services. Ironically, the split between inpatient and outpatient care, coupled with the investment incentives written into the Nixon and Reagan legislation, opened a lucrative new market in outpatient care. Despite claims of patient convenience, the burgeoning outpatient surgeries; diagnostic, birthing, and urgent care centers; and home health services duplicated existing services and further added to excess capacity. Moreover, investor-owned outpatient facilities pulled profitable services away from the hospitals, leaving them with less operating capital to underwrite needed but poorly reimbursed services, such as trauma units and intensive care nurseries.

Throughout the 1970s and 1980s, business was actively involved in the redesign of health care financing. ERISA enabled business to bypass insurance companies altogether. *Purchasing coalitions* were developed, giving business the power of numbers. The coalitions that represented the greatest number of employees typically received the greatest discount from insurance carriers. Since HMOs were highly compatible with purchasing coalitions and tended to offer the lowest premium price, business supported the nascent HMOs.

Business intervention caused profit-protecting adjustments within the insurance sector. Petitioning for deregulation legislation, insurers abandoned the traditional community rating for experience rating. These differential rates let insurers cover their costs on high-risk patients, or even avoid them altogether. With each market segment theoretically paying its own way, the old, the sick, people with risky genetics and pre-existing conditions, and those in dangerous occupations paid the highest premiums or were simply redlined.

Insurers also tightened the rates they paid to providers and increased the co-payments and deductibles they charged patients. Indemnity insurers and Medicare continued the practice of *balance billing*. Prohibited by HMOs, balance billing is another method of shifting costs to the patient. With balance billing, the provider charges the patient for the difference between his or her customary fee and the amount paid by the insurance company.

The multiple, disparate cost-control measures simply reinforced profit-protecting reactions within each stakeholder group, and the number of Americans without insurance began to rise. The provider sector reacted, too, with profit-protecting adjustments. Seeking wealthier insured patients, many providers moved to the suburbs or closed their practices to uninsured patients. Some for-profit hospitals avoided the uninsured by closing their emergency and obstetrics departments, leaving the cost of indigent and Medicaid care to public-funded and religious hospitals.

THE CORPORATIZATION OF HEALTH CARE

At the same time business was involving itself in health care financing, Wall Street was investing in health care. The combination of federal investment dollars and health care's generous profit margins made health care attractive to investors. This attractiveness, augmented by the merger mania and deregulation that signified the 1980s, reinforced the growth of investor-owned, national chains of for-profit hospitals, nursing homes, physician management corporations, and outpatient services, as well as insurance companies that rapidly morphed into managed care organizations.

In less than two decades, investment incentives shifted health care away from solo practitioners and nonprofit organizations to corporate conglomerates. So profound is the corporate influence on the management practices of health care that the only difference between the for-profits and the nonprofits is that the nonprofits do not pay taxes and the for-profits return a portion of their revenue to stockholders.

Managing the business of health care required additional layers of bureaucracy, more overseers, and sophisticated administrators. Also, new regulations and the new paperwork required legions of record-keeping personnel and generated new industries of consultants and computer software programs. This greatly increased the number of health care employees, as lawyers, accountants, lobbyists, consultants, computer and marketing specialists, and other nonclinical persons found jobs in health care. Between 1970 and 1991, the number of health care administrators in the United States increased by 697 percent, compared to a 129 percent increase in clinical personnel.[13]

Corporatization rationalized health care. Managed by the numbers, diseases are construed as product lines; treatments are mechanized; unprofitable diseases, services, and patients are dropped from production. Highly trained personnel are replaced with cheaper, more narrowly qualified personnel (for instance, registered nurses are replaced with patient care technicians). In general, human beings—patients or personnel—are perceived as economic statistics to be ratcheted up or down in order to increase efficiency.

For two decades, business costs rose less sharply, but corporatization did not contain total health care costs. Instead, the number of Americans without access to care increased dramatically, and costs rose almost tenfold. Between 1970 and 1990, total health expenditures rose from $74.3 billion to $696.6 billion. During the same period, Medicare's costs rose from $7.2 billion to $109 billion, while Medicare enrollment merely doubled.

The elderly have been especially vulnerable to cost shifting. In 1972, the elderly spent 10.6 percent of their income on health care, which rose to 16.2 percent in 1984, and 17.1 percent in 1991.[14] Medi-Gap premiums, insurance that supplements Medicare, plus direct out-of-pocket costs for co-pays, deductibles, and uncovered services—especially drugs—account for the bulk of the increased spending. Researchers estimate that if the current trend continues, by 2025, the elderly will spend about 30 percent of their income on health care, and 60 percent of their income will be spent by those in poor health without Medi-Gap coverage.[15]

Since the 1970s, providers and payers have discovered ways to capitalize on federal cost containment policies. The net effect: Costs continue to rise but are redistributed, primarily to patients. Patients assumed more of the costs of health care, paying about 30 percent of all medical costs out of their own pockets. Between 1970 and 1990, the average per-person expenditure rose sharply. Using 1992 data, Steuerle estimated the average expenditure per household at $8,000 per year. Of this, about a third is direct, out-of-pocket expenses. The other two-thirds are indirect: taxes that finance various public programs, which range from Medicare to pharmaceutical research, and wages lost to insurance premiums. In real dollars, American taxpayers contribute almost as much to health care as many governments spend on national health care for their entire population.[16]

Rather than containing costs, economic growth was reinforced by the market incentives championed by the Nixon and Reagan-Bush administrations and is further reinforced by the pro-corporation economic policies—deregulation, privatization, tax cuts, and tort reform—of George W. Bush. Pursuing efficiency rather than effectiveness, everyone raises prices and the fallout is harmful to people and to health care itself. More and more businesses can't afford to purchase health insurance for their employees; tax cuts make it more difficult for the poor to qualify for Medicaid; fewer providers are willing to care for Medicare, Medicaid, and charity patients; competing for insurance dollars, doctors and hospitals duplicate services; and payers invent new ways to avoid unprofitable people and services. As a result, costs continue to soar and the market continues to expand. Health care's traditional altruistic values have given way to corporate values. Frightened away from so-called socialized medicine, Americans ended up with corporate medicine.

MANAGED CARE

By the time Clinton was elected president, most Americans knew someone who had lost his health insurance, who had been denied health care because she couldn't pay for it, or who went without filling a prescription or put off minor surgery because he couldn't afford it. Unsurprisingly, soaring costs and the public's fears made health care reform a major issue in the 1992 presidential election. Although the Clinton plan would have given all Americans access to an affordable, basic package of health care benefits, it failed to get through Congress. By the end, the 1,364-page bill had neither public nor political support. Reform defaulted to managed care since it was already in place and seen by many politicians and reformers alike as *the* cost containment solution.[17]

Managed care is the outgrowth of Nixon's HMO legislation. Proposed by Paul Ellwood Jr., a Minneapolis physician, as a corporate alternative to fee-for-service, high-technology, sick care, the HMO featured prepayment financing, utilization review, and prevention. Its goal was to keep people healthy. The availability of federal investment capital served to make HMOs a private initiative rather than another government-funded bureaucracy. Also, the putative emphasis on keeping people healthy, which would be attained through screening, prevention, and early intervention, made HMOs an attractive solution.

Ellwood's model was the renowned Kaiser-Permanente, a vertically integrated organization in which physicians, hospitals, and insurance are incorporated into one coherent whole. The highly respected model, however, rapidly devolved into a variety of organizations collectively known as *managed care*, a term used interchangeably with HMOs. However, the typical managed care organization is not a vertically integrated organization but a retrofitted insurance carrier, which pays for and manages a broad range of health care goods and services for a defined, or covered, population.

Essentially, managed care is a three-way contract—among the purchaser, the managed care organization, and a network of providers—that integrates the delivery and financing of health care. Prepayment financing and utilization controls distinguish it from indemnity insurance.

The purchaser—usually an employer or the government—negotiates with the managed care organization to pay for and manage the health care of that group of patients. Premiums are risk adjusted. Since purchasers shop for the best health plan at the most affordable price, large employers and purchasing coalitions usually get better prices through volume discounts. Small employers typically pay hefty rates.

The *health plan*, or *covered benefits*, is the slate of services, procedures, specialists, hospitals, doctors, and even ambulance companies the managed care organization will pay for. More expensive plans typically cover a wider range of services and charge lower co-pays and deductibles. Plans vary widely, however, and most policies have substantial exclusion causes. For instance, infertility studies and bone marrow transplants are often not covered. Preauthorization and other restrictions control utilization, although patients can demand services not covered by their health plan. For instance, they can demand to see a specialist who is not in the network, but they must pay for all uncovered services out of their own pocket.

Managed care organizations contract with a select network of providers—a limited panel of hospitals, pharmacies, physician groups, and others who provide the services to enrolled members. Contracts typically include utilization, quality oversight, and payment controls. That providers share the financial risk is probably managed care's most salient feature. The most risk-sharing form of payment is known as *capitation*. Under capitation, providers are paid a fixed monthly fee to take care of the patients enrolled in a particular health plan. Providers receive this predetermined fee regardless of how little or how much the members use the providers' services.

Not all providers are paid by capitation. Payment methods vary, ranging from capitation to DRGs to discounted fee-for-service rates. Scarce specialists, such as neurosurgeons, often contract for the traditional fee-for-service reimbursement. To induce efficiency, however, all contracts typically include cash bonuses for keeping utilization below a certain threshold and guarantee financial penalties to those who are over budget.

During the mid-1990s, managed care helped to contain health care costs. Cost containment was achieved by reducing payments to providers and by controlling patients' access to expensive hospital care and specialists. Providers, however, have made profit-protecting adjustments to managed care's financing. Primary care physicians do more of what is rewarded, such as discharging patients early from the hospital, treating patients themselves rather than making referrals to specialists, and substituting technologically intensive procedures for less-lucrative interventions. Providers also perform fewer activities associated with financial penalties, which means *deselecting* patients with high costs, poor compliance, or poor response to treatment; and they significantly limit the number of Medicaid and charity patients they treat.

Competition means winners and losers, and the pharmaceutical industry was the economic winner of the 1990s, for pharmaceutical benefits reinforce both demand and supply. Before managed care, drugs were priced at what people typically could afford out of pocket. Once a significant proportion of the public has pharmaceutical benefits, drug companies peg their prices to the deeper pockets of the insurance industry. Supply increases as new and more expensive drugs are pulled into the market, because the payer picks up most of the tab. Demand increases because co-payments seemingly cap the out-of-pocket costs of patients with drug benefits. Payers compensate—by raising premium rates across the board. Those without drug benefits are hurt the worst as they pay the full, soaring retail price.

The patient, health care's reason to be, is the unfortunate loser in this competitive game of economic musical chairs. The news is full of managed care stories, of patients refused necessary treatment, of patients charged for an emergency room (ER) visit because their chest pain turned out to be indigestion rather than a heart attack, of patients denied psychiatric admissions that ended as suicides-homicides. The media is also replete with stories of patients who have had eleven primary care physicians in five years because of health plan changes, of patients who couldn't afford a new plan when their HMO pulled out of their geographic area, of small employers who can no longer afford health insurance premiums, of 933,000 elderly and disabled patients who may not have been able to find or afford a new plan after their HMO pulled out of the Medicare program on January 1, 2001.

Despite its entrepreneurial promises of efficiency and competition, managed care did not contain total health care costs. Between 1990 and 2000, total health care costs rose from $696.6 billion to $1.3 trillion. Premium costs, which were relatively flat during most of the 1990s, jumped 10 percent to 30 percent nationwide, benefits were trimmed, and co-pays and deductibles were increased. The number of uninsured rose from 36 million to 44 million, and the percentage of Americans who had health insurance through their jobs fell from 67 percent to 60 percent because employers couldn't afford the premiums or workers couldn't afford their firms' coverage.[18]

Managed care neither keeps people healthier nor reduces health care costs. Instead, managed care reinforces a cascade of reactions; payers protect their profits by avoiding sick people and unprofitable geographic areas, second-guessing doctors, limiting covered services, and shifting more costs to providers and patients.

Moreover, managed care's elaborate central administrative system and massive utilization review staffs are inordinately expensive, as are the dollars needed to pay stockholder dividends and the multimillion-dollar salaries of some of its CEOs. Its management, marketing, and overhead costs account for approximately 33 cents per dollar of claims paid, significantly more than the 2 cents Medicare pays or the 3 cents the Canadian system pays for the same line items.[19]

THE HIGH COSTS OF ECONOMIC REFORM

That patients pay more and receive less are the so-called cost savings of economic reform. In the name of competition, economic growth is pursued through the elimination of unprofitable services and unprofitable people, and by increasing the patients' out-of-pocket costs.

Seen solely through the lens of economics, health care is simply another process to produce capital, and human beings are another raw material consumed in the pursuit of profit. Although good for business, the price to humans is dear. Forty-three million Americans—the already sick, the poor, people of color, unorganized labor, and children—are excluded from the system. So are the estimated 40 million working Americans—one in four adults—who didn't fill a prescription, get a recommended test, or see a doctor because they couldn't afford it. Their loss of access is the cost savings extracted by untempered economic reform.

Quality is also compromised. Many health care employees are frustrated and frightened. The grinding pace of production leaves no time for reflection. Errors increase exponentially: wrong legs are amputated, wrong people disconnected from ventilators, wrong medicines given. In the heat of cutthroat competition, care is delayed and denied. Yet the market is doing, and has been doing, what it is designed to do: provide unlimited economic growth.

MARKET FAILURE

In an economic game, profits grow by raising prices, entering new markets, and/or by reducing production costs. Since the 1950s, health care has used a combination of these three methods to amass an economic value that now represents 14 percent of the GDP in the United States. Although the various groups of players blame one another for mismanagement and waste, what one group calls waste is simply another's profits. It is not an accident that health care costs rose with Medicare and rose again with managed care.

Because health care is financed within the constraints of our market economy, there is much to be learned from reviewing the highlights of the recent history of health care financing. After all, isn't it often suggested that health care be allowed to respond to the checks and balances of the marketplace? Doesn't laissez-faire ideology suggest that market excesses will correct themselves, provided that neither the government nor regulators interfere with the market's self-correcting mechanisms?

A purely competitive market is characterized by three ideals: ideal competition, ideal information, and ideal price. Ideal competition assumes a marketplace with a large number of competing producers and free, or unrestricted, entry for new producers. Consumers have complete information about the price and quality of the product. There is one optimal price—the equilibrium of production costs and price, cued by supply and demand.

Health care inherently violates these ideals. On the supply side, entry isn't free. One can't simply open a hospital, start an HMO, or say "I'm a doctor." On the demand side, consumers don't have complete information about price and quality, nor can patients order their own MRI or prescribe their own antibiotics. Also, employers, not patients, typically purchase health plans, and physicians generally determine how much and what kind of care the patient receives.

In a pure market, competition disciplines *all* players equally. But the health care market is inherently and significantly different from a purely free market. In a free market, the most efficient way to make money is to reduce production costs, but in health care reducing production costs means avoiding sick and poor people, limiting care, and avoiding costly services—behaviors simply contradictory to the purpose of health care. Because those most in need of health care's services are the most costly, all players can never be disciplined equally. Therefore, attempts make health care more marketlike simply increase opportunism and inefficiencies and make the system more dysfunctional overall.

Paul Feldstein claims that the piecemeal nature of health care legislation and regulation is rational and essentially does what it was intended to do.[20] Its purpose is to serve a particular group's economic self-interest at other groups' expense. This reinforces a give-and-take between self-interest groups and politicians. Those groups who contribute the most toward politicians' election receive the power of the state to achieve their own self-interests. That is why health care legislation and regulation often have more to do with benefiting special interest groups than with the efficient use of scarce resources or what is best for the nation's health.

As thirty years of market reforms have demonstrated, the starting point for controlling costs is not to tinker with policies to make health care more efficient. Instead, the starting point is to ask publicly, "What is the purpose of health care? What is best for the nation's health?" Once the answers are in place, we can derive methods that truly make the most efficient use of scarce resources.

CHAPTER 2

Review of Systems

> The problems of today can't be solved with the same thinking that created them.
>
> Albert Einstein

Why are health care's problems so intractable? For decades, policy makers and power brokers have tampered with the structure of health care—changing access here, modifying reimbursement schemes there, applying new layers of bureaucracy everywhere. Despite their best analytical thinking, the fixes tend to make things worse. Costs continue to rise; quality and access continue to deteriorate.

We have the most expensive health care system in the world, but it ranks thirty-seventh worldwide in keeping people healthy, and 43 million Americans are without health insurance. We don't see these three facts as interrelated. Even when the problems with the health care system affect us personally—such as when breast cancer bankrupts our sister's family, or our retired neighbor has to seek part-time work to cover the cost of his prescription drugs, or our HMO refuses to pay for ER care because our chest pain turned out to be indigestion instead of a heart attack—we don't recognize these problems as the result of forty years of piecemeal solutions. Incremental or piecemeal solutions cannot solve health care's problems. Cost, quality, and access aren't separate problems; fixing any one automatically impacts the other two.

When health care doesn't match our expectations or when the "improvements" make things worse, we cite poor planning or ineffective leadership, or we blame our favorite scapegoat. As a society, Americans tend to intervene where a problem is most noticeably visible rather than address the source of the problem. It's a bad habit—like treating a fever with aspirin and ignoring an underlying infection. To complicate matters, health care's visible problem differs depending whether one is a doctor, an employer, a patient, or a managed care administrator.

WE UNDERSTAND WHAT WE SEE

U.S. society's current perspective of health care is much like the fable of the blind men and the elephant. The moral of this fable is that each blind man understood the elephant according to what he "saw," and each saw something different. The man nearest the ear said, It moves air like a fan; the one nearest the tusk said, It is sharp like a spear; the man by the flank said, It is massive like a wall; the man next to a leg said, It stands solid like a tree; the man holding the elephant's tail said, No, I think it's like a rope; and the man feeling the elephant's trunk said that the others were all wrong, the elephant was powerful like a python.

We understand what we see. Each blind man saw a different purpose or a different process, depending on what he was touching. The six stakeholder groups—patients, providers, payers, purchasers, purveyors, and politicians—are like the blind men and the elephant. Each group has a different mental image of health care and is largely focused on its particular interests. Protecting its competitive advantage and certain that its perception is the real thing, none of the stakeholder groups can imagine what the others perceive.

The fable here is a metaphor for the past forty years of health care reform, efforts that have turned health care into an economic game. Each stakeholder group is partly right, but is totally wrong in believing that its version describes the whole health care system. The fable also serves as a warning about being closed-minded and advocating a position based on an incomplete understanding of the health care system. Health care is too complex and too specialized for any one group to have all the answers. In systems thinking, the fable is a statement that the whole can't be understood or reduced to its most significant part. Representing the serious misunderstandings that arise from incomplete data, the fable is a reminder that when people understand only a part of the system or attempt to intervene where a problem is most visible, the information significant to changing multiple variables (for instance cost and access) without harming the whole is never seen, which efforts to control costs and subsidize special interests groups have amply demonstrated.

WHAT WE SEE DETERMINES WHAT WE DO

This book is about seeing things whole, because what we see determines what we do. If Americans are to escape the liabilities of piecemeal reform, which persists in making health care an economic game, then we need to see that the current popular concerns—the affordability of pre-scription drugs for seniors, and the affordability of out-of-pocket costs of health care services and health insurance for low- and middle-income families—are, in fact, tied to deeper core issues.

Paradoxically, the most effective way to control health care costs is by addressing the deeper issues of today—such as chronic disease and end-of-life care, the ethics of health care's unhealthy dependence on expensive technology, the social and environmental determinants of health, the depersonalization of care, and the gross disparities in health status and health care that fall along ethnic and economic lines. These core issues can't be addressed piecemeal or at the covered population level. In fact, these seemingly intractable issues can be resolved only if Americans find the courage to take off their blindfolds to see health care as a whole.

While this book is about seeing the whole health care system, it is also about the processes of taking off our blindfolds. Taking off our blindfolds signifies more than seeing what other stakeholders see; it's about escaping the blinders of fear, ignorance, and selfishness that have prevented us from discovering a more healthy health care system.

AN OVERVIEW OF THE WHOLE

From a postmodern perspective, health care is both a part and a whole. Health care is not an independent system. It doesn't exist in a vacuum, in other words, but is a system within a nested hierarchy of systems: the individual self, health care, our market economy, and an overarching worldview. Of these forces, the worldview is the most influential.

To see this nested hierarchy more clearly, imagine a set of Russian dolls, the wooden kind that opens to reveal an ever-smaller doll (Figure 2.1). Each doll is both a part and a whole. Nested together, each doll is merely a part of a larger whole. When the set is taken apart, each doll is whole by itself. Each doll represents one system.

In this analogy, the smallest doll represents the individual self, the recipient of health care's output. The next doll is the health care system, and the third doll represents our market economy. Containing all of this is the largest and least-visible doll, the worldview.

WORLDVIEWS

Because everything that we do begins as some kind of thought, removing blindfolds begins by acknowledging the deepest thought that informs our actions. This seems obvious, but very few people are actually aware of their thoughts on a moment-by-moment basis. As a result, our actions are auto-matic, based on how society has conditioned us to think about health care.

The most deeply embedded conditioning is known as a worldview. Worldviews are the mental conditioning through which we see the world.

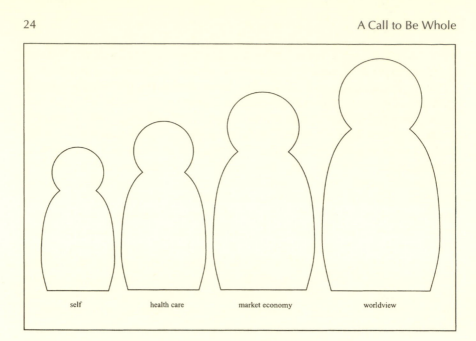

Figure 2.1 Health Care Is Both a Part and a Whole

Formed from thought—powerful, overarching beliefs, deeply imbedded
in a culture that explain the laws and architecture of life itself—worldviews are more than theoretical foundations from which society's norms
and social institutions are derived, for worldviews prescribe the way we
learn to identify ourselves as embodied persons and embody that identity.
Worldviews inform our behavior, shape our social and civic relationships,
and determine our beliefs, including beliefs about sickness, health, and
death.

   We are usually unaware of our worldview, however, because we take it
for granted. Like water to fish, the dominant worldview is so integral to
the functioning of society that it is indispensable and unacknowledged.
It's invisible. The more powerful the worldview, the more invisible it is,
and the less likely we are to connect our behavior to it, and the more automatic our actions.

   The other reason we are usually unaware is that worldviews are self-
sealing. In other words, each worldview uses its own information to prove
its logic and uses its own logic to validate its information. Moreover,
worldviews establish our scientific exemplars. These exemplars determine how a problem is framed; the technology used to investigate the
problem; the kinds of data that are valid and important—and the kinds
that we disregard—and the logic used in fashioning our solutions. For
instance, fearing socialized medicine, Americans simply accept as real the

arbitrary linkage between health insurance and employment, accept universal health insurance as anathema, and then are surprised when tinkering with health care's reimbursement mechanisms doesn't bring down costs but instead raises the numbers of uninsured. Similarly, the U.S. medical community's using its hegemony over what constitutes "scientific,"—usually without examining the evidence—to dismiss other healing systems as unscientific is another example of the self-sealing power of a worldview.

The self-sealing nature of one's worldview is the reason why a Navajo shaman, an allopathic medical doctor, and an Ayurvedic physician each sees different symptoms and recommends different treatments, even though they are looking at the very same patient. Information that is valid to one may be irrelevant to the others. Which goes to prove, when our worldviews differ, we literally can't see another's point of view.

Because they are taken for granted and self-sealing, worldviews remain out of sight—until they begin to fail, which they inevitably do. A sharp rise in the number of exceptions to the rules and the accumulation of exceptions to the exceptions are sure signs of a failing worldview. Exceptions arise because scientific exemplars will eventually raise issues not resolvable within the constraints of the worldview. Thus, a worldview sows the seeds of its own destruction. Albert Einstein put it another way, saying the problems of today couldn't be solved with the same thinking that created them.

Failure is a blessing in disguise, however. Failure forces us to be aware of what was once a taken-for-granted worldview. This is a good thing, since we can't fully perceive new ideas without understanding the limitations of the old. For example, the movement of signals along nerve fibers can't be explained by Newtonian exemplars but is readily explained by quantum mechanics. Failure means our knowledge is evolving. With the insights to transcend previous misunderstanding, we can create something more coherent, and that is a blessing, indeed.

It is not a coincidence that Americans are currently engaged in a debate about how to reduce health care costs. We're finally feeling the failure of modern assumptions.

CAUGHT BETWEEN TWO COMPETING WORLDVIEWS

Every system of healing emerges from its society's prevailing worldview. In any culture, health care exists within certain moral and technological frameworks, and it serves certain socioeconomic functions. Because it is the nature of systems of healing to deal with crisis, *dis-ease*, and the disruption of what is considered normal, every health care system is highly sensitive to shifts in the deep beliefs that organize society and inform our behavior. In a nutshell, we are living in a conflict-laden time when the once dominant worldview, the modern worldview, is no longer taken for granted, but the postmodern worldview, the source of the significant scientific advancements of the twentieth century, is not taken for granted either. That is to say, the U.S. health care system is caught between two competing worldviews: the modern worldview, which organizes the current health care system, and the postmodern worldview, which gives us a radically different understanding of systems and a holistic understanding of health.

Each worldview presents a very different understanding of systems in general and of health care in particular. Figure 2.2 illustrates the differences. Notice that the modern worldview is enveloped by the postmodern one. This shows that our knowledge is evolving. It does not indicate that modern exemplars are passé; that would be throwing out the baby with the bathwater. The figure simply indicates that we can understand the limitations of a Newtonian view of space, time, matter, and causality from the vantage point of quantum physics. We know a lot more about the organization of life than we did 300 years ago—and there's more still to be discovered, as the arrows pointing outward depict.

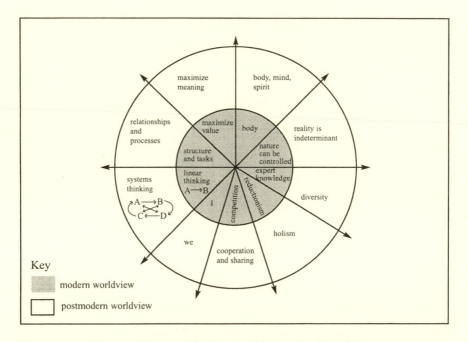

Figure 2.2 Differences between Modern and Postmodern Worldviews
Source: Adapted from Linda Ellinor & Glenda Gerard (1998). *Dialogue: Rediscovering the Transforming Power of Conversation.* New York: John Wiley & Sons, p. 45.

THE MODERN WORLDVIEW

In the sixteenth and seventeenth centuries, the world became demystified. Before then, humans were enmeshed in nature and the supernatural. Early healers were typically priests, shamans, and folk healers, and sickness was attributed to forces of nature and the supernatural. Sickness was thought to be caused by such things as evil spirits, broken taboos, "unclean" persons, and bad weather and was typically treated with the use of charms and rituals, which were augmented by roots and herbs and whatever else was at the disposal of the early healers.

To demystify the world, men such as René Descartes, Isaac Newton, and John Locke invoked a new power, the power of human knowledge. A new way of knowing emerged, which we refer to as the scientific method. Here was born the dualistic philosophy of Descartes, a philosophy that separated spirit from matter and the mind from the body. Newtonian physics presented the universe as if it were a mechanical clock and led us to believe that subject and object are separate and that we could control nature of we could reduce it to its smallest component.

As the world was demystified, power shifted from the divine right of kings and priests to those with expert knowledge. The self was established as a separate entity, which Locke later imbued with inalienable rights, and utilitarian ethics gained sovereignty. Positing that the right action in any circumstance is that which produces the greatest good for the greatest number, its basic principle is to maximize value.

Modernity's gift to the world is the differentiation of mind, body, and spirit. Insight into the laws of nature and mathematical modeling—the twin engines of scientific discovery—drove the ascendancy of the natural sciences and economics. With its focus on matter, the modern worldview assumes (1) that nature can be controlled if reduced to its smallest component, the atom; (2) that objective, or "hard scientific," data are more valid than subjective thoughts and feelings; and (3) that technology is value-free and morally neutral.

In accordance with classical physics, the modern worldview posits that the parts are primary and the system is generated by their interaction. Its exemplars present a reductionistic, materialistic, mechanistic view of systems, and of life itself. Accordingly, we think linearly; that is, we assume things behave according to a fixed simple and direct relationship: A causes B, B causes C, and so forth. Moreover, the reductionistic understanding of nature fosters discipline-based thinking, isolating each stakeholder group in its own knowledge box. Once within the box, no group can see the whole.

THE POSTMODERN WORLDVIEW

In contrast, the newer, postmodern worldview posits that a system can't be reduced to its most significant part. Instead, the whole is primary and possesses properties and qualities that can't be deduced from its parts. Associated with quantum physics and Einstein's theory of relativity, the postmodern worldview presents a new set of concepts regarding space, time, matter, and causality. Its exemplars include holism, relativity, self-organization, and nonlinear relationships.

Around the middle of the twentieth century, Ludwig Berthalanffy and other pioneers of this revolutionary point of view posited that systems are more fully understood in light of internal *and* external relationships. In other words, the influence of outside contexts is as important to a system's structure and function as is the operation of its internal parts. Since the 1950s, this worldview has steadily gained acceptance in the scientific community as it became apparent that a holistic worldview could better explain the complexities of biology and social sciences and better support developments in computer technology and artificial intelligence.

Developments in subatomic physics, chaos theory, and fractal mathematics have also strengthened the postmodern worldview. Briefly, the postmodern worldview assumes that matter, information, and energy are different aspects of the same phenomenon; nothing in this world occurs in isolation; no thing is permanent; and reality is more than the material world.

Holism posits that a system's behavior is best understood by virtue of complex interdependent relationships among (1) the elements that generate the system, (2) the processes inside the system, and (3) the other systems whose outputs the system receives in the form of material and information. Holism's metaphor is a goldfish bowl. Water, fish, and plants are autonomous systems. Together they form a complex whole, existing by virtue of their interdependent relationships. Each system depends upon the inputs of other systems and needs other systems to receive its outputs. Directly or indirectly affecting one another, each system behaves the way it does because of the actions of the other two. To change one system is to change them all; each system needs the others to be itself.

WRONG ANSWERS TO WRONG QUESTIONS

Health care's rising costs and diminishing returns are both significant issues and make plenty of headlines; however, costs are what we see. By continuing to narrowly focus on insurance and drugs costs, or on health care's costs in general, we miss the important connections between cost, quality, and access—the connections that now make health care an economic game.

We are, so to speak, ignoring the whole elephant, or acting from the modern worldview. Our minds see health care as an independent system, disconnected from the beliefs, values, and rules of our market economy;

and our minds reduce health care to its most "significant" part, costs. Constrained by the way modernity frames the problem, we continue to tinker with costs. As a result, we either attempt to make health care more efficient, or we subsidize the marginalized. Managed care is an example of the former approach and Medicare, an example of the later. Now the George W. Bush administration is tentatively looking at various proposals to subsidize drug costs for Medicare recipients and health insurance costs for low-income workers.

The problem is that tinkering with costs simply pours more money into health care. Pouring money into the system is not the same as turning off the economic spigot. Pouring money doesn't halt the economic gaming. Although it may keep the marginalized in the game a little longer, it doesn't stop the waste and opportunism or improve quality.

Whether at the policy level or at the public-opinion-poll level, attempts to control costs as the only variable will give us the wrong answers to the wrong questions, consistently. Tinkering is acting with incomplete data. Tinkering is the cliché garbage in, garbage out.

TO ASK THE RIGHT QUESTIONS IS TO OBTAIN THE RIGHT ANSWERS

Paradoxically, the most effective way to contain cost is not to tinker inside the health care system but to begin with the question, "What is best for the nation's health?" It's a significant, overarching question, and one that can eventually lead us to an economic shut-off valve, as the next four chapters will show.

Because health is something health care produces, asking what is best for the nation's health forces us (1) to define health care's product, or identify the attributes of health, and (2) to decide whose health actually concerns us. Right now, Americans do not have one clear and consistent understanding of health and disagree whether the purpose of health care is to maintain the health of single individuals, covered populations, or Americans as a whole.

If health care reform is to result in an efficient and effective system, then whose health and which attributes of health are we concerned with, anyway? For example, it's not uncommon for senior citizens on Medicare to have from $400 to $700 a month in drug costs, but does every senior need every medical intervention, no matter how uncertain or small the benefit may be? It may be good defensive medicine, but we've got to ask ourselves, is it really beneficial to that senior, or to the rest of society, for a seventy-five-year-old with diabetes to be on an expensive cholesterol-lowering medication? Are there preexisting conditions for which or an age at which it's foolish to attempt to prevent heart attacks and heart disease? What about the forty-five-year-old who is a family's primary wage earner and can't afford the cholesterol-lowering drugs? Should the government subsidize him or her as well? In the case of our seventy-five-year-old, would it be more sensible to subsidize something else, such as help with grocery shopping, that might be more important to his or her health? What's more, is it fair for the government to subsidize the drug costs of seniors and not subsidize the insurance costs of workers who can't afford health insurance? When do we say *enough?*

Are we concerned about the health status of individuals or the whole population? What does "health" mean to a seventy-five-year-old? Does it mean the same to a twenty-five-year-old, a ninety-five-year-old, a premature infant, or someone with a disability or a chronic disease? Who is responsible to decide? Unless we know whose health and which attributes of health concern us, anyway, none of the questions in this and the preceding paragraph—*questions that are directly related to health care costs*—can be reliably answered.

Improving health care's efficiency and effectiveness begins with asking the right questions. To have the right answers, we have to ask the right questions, and to ask the right questions we have to know how health care is organized.

THE ORGANIZATION OF HEALTH CARE

Every system of healing is a social system generated by human thought and organized according to a society's prevailing worldview. To see this organization more clearly, imagine health care as a cultural box (Figure 2.3). Its walls are formed from society's answers to four age-old questions that have informed all systems of healing since the beginning of time: What is health? What is care? How much is enough? and Who is responsible? These questions are the subjects of the next four chapters.

The answers to these questions generate a dynamic configuration of patients, healers, scientific theories and technologies, ethnical and social values, and economic and political power. This is the basic pattern, regardless of how primitive or sophisticated we deem a society's health care system. Although every system involves this configuration, the configuration is not static but shifts with the tides of time and human thought.

No health care system is inherently right or wrong. (However, productive health care systems do produce the expected product—health—without wasting resources.) Even systems that seem foreign or primitive are not a hodgepodge of meaningless rites. Instead, the basic pattern is found in each, influenced by its society's understanding of the human body and whether sickness is a merely a personal concern or a societal concern that represents a rent in the social fabric. The moral value ascribed to sickness, the influence of science and technology, society's mode of production, and the value of labor also contribute to health care's basic pattern.

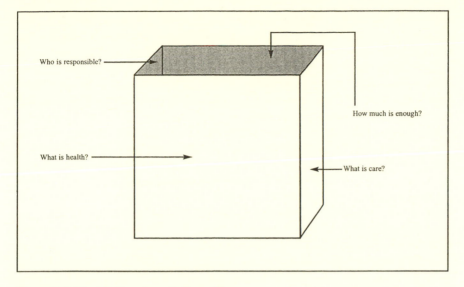

Figure 2.3 Health Care As a Cultural Box

These influences, known as cultural variables because they vary by society and historical period, inform and shape our answers to the four questions. Moreover, that the variables are derived from the prevailing worldview means that health care is compatible with and connected to the other social institutions, such as education, religion, economics, and politics.

The Russian doll analogy of Figure 2.1 is useful here. Health care is packed inside an economic system that is packed again inside a specific worldview. It is only in our imagination that we can separate these parts from the whole we call health care. Even harder to grasp, perhaps, is that much of health care's pattern is nothing more than the product of spoken thought.

THE MODERN U.S. HEALTH CARE SYSTEM

The contemporary U.S. health care system is firmly grounded in the modern worldview, in which reality is reduced to the laws of nature, and the body is perceived as a mechanical entity with interchangeable parts. Basically, health care is medical care, which is profit-driven, individually focused, reduced to drugs and surgery, physician authorized, and fragmented by medical specialty. Health is the absence of disease; disease is caused by a single biological variable—germs, genes, or trauma; and the physician is responsible for producing health. Any notion of enough is moot, because materialism encourages Americans to believe that technology—if not this generation, the next—can control nature, defeat death and disability, and delay aging. It is a linear production model in which sickness → drugs + surgery → cure.

Until about 1970, our health care system worked fairly well. Now, financial experts with master's degrees in business administration challenge medical authority. Critics point to rising costs and diminishing returns, the inequities of access, and health care's inadequacy in caring for people with chronic diseases and life-threatening illnesses. Researchers point out the ineffectiveness of high-tech medicine for treating social and environmental problems, such as child abuse and lead poisoning, that are handed off to providers, and health care's ineffectiveness in caring for the population's health. Finally, the public wants more than their physicians can provide and has turned to myriad forms of alternative care.

Our health care system is unproductive. That much, everyone agrees. The problem is, all Americans don't see the same health care system. Answers to our four questions vary depending upon whether one is a patient, a provider, or a payer. To further complicate matters, Americans don't agree whether health care is a commodity for those who can afford its price, or a social good necessary for the nation's well-being.

UNPACKING HEALTH CARE

Because our thinking determines what we see and do, the purpose of this book is to inquire into the thought that generates our health care system. If we don't expose the thinking, then our actions remain automatic and we are destined to repeat and reinforce the factors that make the modern system dysfunctional. In short, we make things worse. That is the lesson of managed care reform, in which specific costs and profits were merely shifted as overall costs continued to soar.

Making things worse is the reason Americans fear another round of sweeping changes to health care, according to a 2002 public opinion poll by National Public Radio (NPR), the Kaiser Family Foundation and Harvard University's Kennedy School of Government. The poll found that 57 percent of Americans said major changes are needed, but only 23 percent believe health care to be so dysfunctional that it should be completely rebuilt.[1] This is counter to polls conducted in 1992, when the majority of Americans thought health care should be completely rebuilt.

Paradoxically, the only way to escape the vicious cycle of rising costs and diminishing returns is through *inquiry*, not through piecemeal financial and quality change. Seeing the thought that generates the health care system is the same as asking the right questions, or as taking off the blindfolds so we can see the whole. Similar to reverse engineering or archaeological excavations, inquiry refers to unpacking the nested hierarchy of systems to which health care belongs.

To inquire is to expose layers of thought—scientific theories, ethical and social values, and economic and political philosophies—that generate the American health care system. In simple terms, to inquire is to connect thought with its manifestation. Inquiry is an examination of one's deepest beliefs against the backdrop of others' beliefs and reveals why we believe what we believe about health, care, responsibility, and enough. To inquire is to expose, and to expose is to become aware of, and because our actions always originate as thought, exposing our thinking connects our thought to our actions and makes us aware of the effect our actions have on other people. To inquire is to take off the blindfolds.

SYSTEMS THINKING

Systems thinking is a term that refers to the postmodern understanding of systems.[2] In contrast to modernity, which organizes information in terms of parts, systems thinking organizes information in terms of wholes. It is a conceptual framework for explaining complex interactions, for seeing wholes *and* interacting parts (as in the goldfish-bowl analogy), for seeing connections rather than structure and tasks, and for seeing patterns and processes.

Like all social systems, health care is a network of relationships in which people and materials interact to form a meaningful whole. Like all systems, health care has definable boundaries, is comprised of identifiable parts that are connected by networks of interlocking feedback loops, receives input from other systems in the form of resources and information, and generates output to the world outside its boundaries. Inputs, outputs, boundaries, and feedback loops are the keys to understanding systems.

In systems language, feedback loops connect the parts. Carrying information and resources, feedback loops are the relationships that hold systems together internally and connect them externally. In everyday language, health care's internal feedback loops are the roles of its various stakeholders and its policies, rules, and regulations. Together, they determine the types and distribution of resources among the stakeholders.

The two types of feedback loops—*reinforcing* and *balancing*—function together much like a series of on and off switches. Reinforcing loops accelerate the processes they turn on; for instance, a snowball rolling downhill or thread emptying off a spool. True to their names, reinforcing loops reinforce growth or decay. In contrast, balancing loops maintain system stability by counteracting, or balancing, the effects of reinforcing loops. For example, the exchanges of O_2 and CO_2 are balancing actions for the fish and plants in the goldfish-bowl analogy.

Boundaries are a kind of barrier. Boundaries include the elements necessary for a system to function and exclude all other elements. Because many systems are interlocking and interdependent, we impose boundaries to tell us where one system ends and another begins. Generally, boundaries begin with an input, typically the product of an external system, and end with an output that is the input for another system. Some boundaries are obvious. Our skin is a natural boundary, separating us from our environment. Other boundaries are more arbitrarily imposed.

The interactions among the elements of any system form an observable pattern, a process repeated over and over in regular and predictable ways. All well-entrenched patterns tend to be stable, and stable systems are productive systems. Incorporating inputs, generating outputs, and conserving resources, productive systems do what they were meant to do without wasting resources. Stable systems are at equilibrium; that is, reinforcing loops are balanced. Equilibrium means the system's energy is at a minimum, a state depicted in chemistry books as a molecule resting in an energy trough. Because it takes additional energy to dislodge a system from its protective energy trough, stable systems tend to resist change.

Still, systems may fail or become dysfunctional. Dysfunctional systems do not do what they were meant to do, or they waste resources because internal or external relationships—or both—are out of balance, or they waste resources because their boundaries are eroding. Because the equilibrium of failing systems is indeed precarious, there is a point at which these systems can quickly tip, or fall apart.

From their study of systems, Peter Senge and other systems theorists have developed a list of guiding principles. Below are a few from Senge's *Fifth Discipline:*

- Today's problems come from yesterday's "solutions."
- Cause and effect are not closely related in space and time.
- Structure influences human behavior.
- To permanently change a system means changing its structure.
- Small changes can produce big results—but the areas of highest leverage are often the least obvious.
- You and the cause of your problems are part of a single system.[3]

Systems thinking shifts our focus from "bad" people, tasks and structure, and linear relationships to processes and nonlinear relationships. It's a perceptual difference, a shift from a static to a dynamic view of systems. It's a switch from modernity's quantitative reductionism to a qualitative, holistic point of view. The significance of a systems mode of inquiry is the ability to see networks of connections, or the dynamic interplay among the system's elements. Thus, we can see the tight connections among quality, costs, and access that make health care today such a deadly game of musical chairs. Having seen the connections, we can direct our efforts to improving the relationships among the whole nested hierarchy, because our health care system is generated as much by its external relationships as by internal relationships.

Unpacking health care includes examining the inputs, outputs, boundaries, and feedback loops for each of the four systems in the nested hierarchy of systems: self, health care, market economy, and worldview.

Process Improvement

Process improvement is the first level of systems thinking and is based on the understanding that performance is a system property; more precisely, process improvement posits that a product cannot be better than its production processes. Generally attributed to W. Edwards Deming,[4] process improvement is part of the quality movement that swept through the manufacturing industry in the 1980s and was brought to health care in 1987 by Donald Berwick, M.D., a pediatrician from Harvard Medical School.[5]

Hospitals and managed care organizations are required by their accrediting agencies to use process improvement principles to become more efficient and to improve the quality of patient care. However, the efforts are entirely local, limited to a single organization or covered population and address pinpoint-specific quality issues, such as reducing the incidence of infection following coronary bypass surgery or increasing the prevalence of mammograms in a covered population.

Process improvement is the first level of inquiry. It is the level to which almost all health care reform efforts are now directed. At this level, inquiry is largely directed toward improving relationships that comprise a single process inside individual organizations and facilities; thus, the focus is on internal processes and feedback loops. While the focus of this first-level inquiry is still largely inside seemingly independent systems, by now some readers are wondering about the network of feedback loops among and between the systems that compose the whole nested hierarchy and the pattern those feedback loops create.

Flood's Holistic Prism

The second level of inquiry focuses on health care's boundaries. More precisely, this level exposes the thought that informs health care's boundaries. Ideally, boundaries include the elements necessary for a system to function productively and exclude everything that is detrimental. Health care's boundaries are the walls in our cultural box analogy.

In our cultural box analogy (Figure 2.3), What is health? is the significant question. Its answer is the load-bearing wall, so to speak. In simple terms, the definition of health informs the four elements that are basic to all health care systems: cause, patient, healer, and remedy. It also means that the answers to the other three questions—What is care? How much is enough? and Who is responsible?—are derived from our answer to What is health? As we will see in the next four chapters, these broad questions expose the cultural variables, thereby enhancing and clarifying our understanding of health care's basic pattern. As shown in Figure 2.4, the cultural variables establish (1) the cause of sickness; (2) the benefits, obligations, and stigmas assigned to patients; (3) the rights, privileges, and responsibilities of the healer; and (4) the goals of healing and the market basket of sanctioned interventions.

Within this second level of inquiry, we ask whether health care's boundaries include the right elements in the right amounts to generate a productive system. Moreover, because boundaries define more than just the *things*—the policies, the technology, the rules, and the roles—that generate health care, we also ask, *who* is in and benefits, and *who* is out and does not,[6] and why?

Because social systems are generated by human thought, boundaries don't occur by accident. They are established by a group of experts whom society has authorized and are based on data that is valid to the experts. Boundary setting is an indication of knowledge power, in other words, and since neither the included beneficiaries nor the excluded losers occur by happenstance, boundary setting is also a moral act.

To understand boundary setting, Robert Lewis Flood, another expert in systems thinking, likens complex systems—such as health care—to a four-sided prism. Depicted in Figure 2.5, each facet reflects one aspect of the system: meaning, effectiveness, efficiency, and fairness.[7]

Briefly, meaning has to do with purpose; effectiveness refers to whether the elements are present so that the system fulfills its purpose; efficiency

Cause of Sickness	Goals of Healing and Sanctioned Interventions
Role of the Healer (Rights, Privileges, and Responsibilities)	Role of the Patient (Benefits, Obligations, and Stigmas)

Figure 2.4 Basic Pattern of Health Care Systems

Meaning	Fairness
Purpose	Knowledge power
Effectiveness	**Efficiency**
Healer, patient, cause, remedy	Conservation of resources

Figure 2.5 Flood's Holistic Prism

has to do with conservation of resources; and fairness refers to the moral use of knowledge power in the establishment of boundaries. Effectiveness and efficiency are ascertained through the first level of inquiry, and fairness refers to a Rawls-like theory of justice. According to John Rawls, a political philosopher, justice is attained if those people who have the power to draw the boundaries choose for everyone else the same as they choose for themselves and their friends.[8]

To envision the importance boundaries have in the formation of a productive health care system, we will return to our analogy of health care as a cultural box (Figure 2.6). Its frame is Flood's four-sided prism: meaning, effectiveness, efficiency, and fairness; and its walls are the answers to the

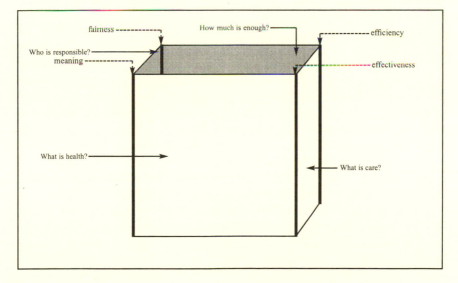

Figure 2.6 A Congruent Health Care System Is One Whose Cover Fits Its Frame

four questions, What is health? What is care? Who is responsible? and How much is enough?

Flood's holistic prism unpacks multiple layers of information, giving us deeper and subtler insights into health care's stability. First, we can see whether our society has one consistent answer to each of the four questions. Multiple answers are like a cell membrane that has begun to leak: the boundary is no longer highly selective in what it allows to enter and leave the cell. Second, we can see whether the four elemental answers are congruent; that is, whether they are not contradictory but, rather, agree with and complement one another. In other words, we'd say the walls of the cultural box fit well together. Third, the prism enables us to see whether the walls coherently fit the frame, and, if it doesn't, we can see where the fit is poor and why. With the health status of Americans ranked thirty-seventh in the world, we know effectiveness is a poor fit.

To unpack, or to see clearly the thought that informs health care's boundaries, is to call attention to the influence cultural variables have in shaping each of the stakeholder group's answers to the four boundary-setting questions. Such exposure not only illuminates the variables but also sheds light on how the variables are used by stakeholders that hold the boundary-setting knowledge power. In this level of unpacking, the feedback loops connecting health care to the other systems in the nested hierarchy are seen. The second level of inquiry also calls attention to society's—and to each stakeholder group's—understanding of meaning, effectiveness, efficiency, and fairness. It's probably no surprise that this inquiry leads us right to health care's organizing worldview. Ironically, such inquiry depends upon a postmodern understanding of systems.

Dialogue

Unpacking the third and deepest level of health care is accomplished through dialogue. Dialogue is to understanding human relationships as systems thinking is to understanding a system's processes. It is a conversation that inquires into our thinking, or a reflexive learning process. In this context, thought is more than the rational intellect. It also includes physical sensations, emotions, perceptions, personality traits, impulses, and desires. In short, dialogue returns us to the source of thought: each person's head and heart. Senge hinted at this with his principle, "You and the cause of your problems are part of a single system."

The source of all our troubles, according to the physicist David Bohm, one of dialogue's leading theorists, is a pervasive incoherence in the process of human thought.[9] Basically, Bohm is saying that we are on automatic pilot. We act according to habit, or a memory-version of reality, which we take for granted as real, rather than acting according to a direct perception of the world around us. We actually don't know what we are doing. Automatic pilot means that we take the concepts that organize our health care system for granted. We have forgotten that these concepts of health care and our beliefs about who should benefit are generated by human thought to serve a certain purpose. When we take something for granted, our thinking has become invisible to us.

Dialogue is about seeing the places in our lives where we simply assume something to be real and operate on automatic pilot. Using dialogue, we become aware of the incoherence in our thinking. Paradoxically, to actually see the incoherence is to have the capacity to see the whole. Metaphorically speaking, to unpack this level of thought is to open our hearts: We can see only what our hearts can hold. Indeed, the phrase "to open our hearts," means to deepen our awareness to this level of inquiry.

At this deepest level of inquiry, we are interested in the structure of our thought, our personal software program, so to speak. At this level, the health care system and its organizing concepts are experienced as processes that inform our self-image and interpersonal relationships. In this space, the thought that informs the quality of human relationships is exposed. It is here that the work of the first two levels of inquiry drops deeper into our awareness. Here, we can finally see more healthy ways to organize the health care system.

MODERNITY'S GIFT AND THE POSTMODERN CHALLENGE

Modernity's gift to the world is the differentiation of mind, body, and spirit. As modernity blossomed and bore fruit, humans could finally do more than petition their gods for help. The elucidation of the laws of nature gave humans some control over nature and fostered the development of technology, making life easier. With the emergence of modern exemplars, creature comforts improved and longevity increased. For the first time, human beings didn't have to worry so much about food, clothing, and shelter.

However, an overreliance on modernity's gifts exacts its own price. We are now feeling that price. Science has led us to overvalue facts and expert opinion and devalue feelings and meaning. The reduction of health to atoms and molecules has fragmented the individual to a collection of biochemical pathways and chromosomes and has fragmented the community to an aggregate of competing individuals. The primacy of the mechanistic worldview leads us to believe that matter is dead; that we can control nature and win the war against disease and aging. With our penchant for objectivity, moral decisions default to quantitative data. Objectivity has become the cliché "it's nothing personal, it's just business," offering the illusion that justice is blind and economic decisions are out of our hands. Committed to our favorite part, we forget about the whole.

A possible gift of postmodern, or holistic thinking, according to Ken Wilber lies in the integration of body, mind, and spirit,[10] something holistic health practitioners have been advocating at the individual level since the early 1980s. From the level of society, however, integration also includes what Wilber refers to as the "big three": I, We, and It. They are Wilber's shorthand for the subjective, or self (I); the intersubjective, or morals (We); and the objective, or science and technology (It). When we think of health care, the health care system is an "it"; those who have insurance are "we," and "I" is self-explanatory. The big three is a sound-byte way of saying that life is whole; don't break it apart for the sake of convenience.

The gift of integration is summarized in two folk sayings: "as above, so below," and "the outside reflects the inside." In systems language, we'd say that human beings and their systems are mutually enfolded. These ideas are scientifically represented by the hologram. Simply speaking, a hologram is a three-dimensional (3D) image made by shining a laser beam on a photographic plate. Its unique feature is that the entire image is completely represented inside every part of itself. We could cut the film into tiny pieces and each piece would still project the whole 3D image.

Health means wholeness, but health care is fractured. Obviously. Not everyone has health insurance or access to health care. Moreover, health care is an aggregate of disparate services, programs, national policies, organizations, competitive special interest groups, and entrepreneurial practices that defy our efforts to see it whole.

To reform the health care system is to heal it. Healing involves the restoration of integrity; to heal means to make whole. That means embracing a worldview that allows us to see wholes rather than championing our favorite part. That in turn leads to repairing dysfunctional relationships within the nested hierarchy of systems. And that depends on finding congruent answers to the four elemental questions and assuring that healer, patient, cause, and remedy are coherent with the frame of Flood's holistic prism.

CHAPTER 3

What Is Health?

What is health? is *the* significant question. As we've seen, the answers to the other three questions—What is care? How much is enough? and Who is responsible?—are derived from our answer to What is health? Moreover, health care's efficiency, effectiveness, and fairness are measured according to the attributes we assign to health.

In our cultural box analogy, What is health? is the load-bearing wall. That Americans have the most expensive health care system in the word but their country ranks thirty-seventh worldwide at keeping people healthy indicates our current definition of health is not able to bear its load. In systems language, we'd say that our current definition of health is inadequate to organize a productive health care system.

INCONSISTENT IMAGES OF HEALTH

But what is health? Words are vehicles for human relationships. Nouns evoke pictures in our heads. To illustrate, the word *elephant* evokes a different mental image than the word *tree*. Unlike the words *elephant* and *tree*, the word *health* does not evoke a consistent image in the minds of either the American public or the experts engaged in health care reform. There is no universally accepted definition of health. There simply isn't a gold standard we can point to and say, This is it. Like *freedom* and *justice*, *health* is difficult to define.

The problem with health care reform is that we rush to tinker with health care costs while assuming everyone has the same idea of health in mind. We don't inquire; we simply assume that health means the same to the insurer as it does to the patient, the same to the young as it does to those with life-threatening disease, the same to you as it does to me. The blind spot in health care reform is that no one sees the same system.

Since about 1850, five definitions for the word *health* have entered the public domain. Their entrances reflect the progression of changing cultural forces. Because each new definition of health did not supersede the old, but merely added to the mix, our society is plagued with multiple, inconsistent definitions of health. Each evokes a different image in the minds of the public and health care's various stakeholders.

Briefly, the definitions come from biomedicine, the World Health Organization (WHO), the Rockefeller Foundation, the wellness ideas of the 1970s, and the concept of community health. Although the basic pattern of health care is always the same, as Figure 2.4 shows, the particulars for each of the four elements of the pattern vary—greatly. Reflecting the progression of changing cultural forces, each definition is distinguished by its own set of concepts regarding the causes of sickness, the object of care and who is eligible for it, the goals of healing and sanctioned methods of treatment, and who has the authority to heal.

Since most Americans are not clear about each definition's distinguishing criteria but have formed a collage from their favorite features, we don't have the same image of health. In fact, when we talk about health and ways to improve health care, we usually are not talking about the same thing at all.

MEDICINE IS THE SCIENCE CONCERNED WITH THE PREVENTION AND CURE OF DISEASE

Fee-for-service health care and its offspring, managed care, are based on the nineteenth-century definition of *medicine:* "the science of diagnosing, treating, curing, and preventing disease."[1] Most medical schools still use this definition.

The word *medicine* refers to one specific type of healing: biomedicine. Biomedicine goes by many different names: scientific medicine, allopathic medicine, traditional medicine, and acute care medicine. What Americans call health care is actually biomedicine, a name that corporate marketers changed in the 1980s to health care to present the public with an upbeat image of perfection and unlimited consumer possibilities. Health's images of youth, happiness, virility, longevity, and beauty are more enticing than the medical images of sickness and suffering.

Biomedicine is the grandchild of modernity. Evolving with the development of classical physics and chemistry, biomedicine presumes a reductionistic, materialistic, deterministic view of human beings. In biomedicine, the Cartesian view of man as machine, constructed from interchangeable parts, still prevails. Disease is an objective, *physical* phenomenon and is defined as a molecular breakdown caused by one specific vector—be it microbes, faulty genes, toxins, or trauma. Reductionism and materialism—the notion that all events inside the body can be explained by the laws of nature (that is, of classical physics and chemistry)—are reinforced by linear thinking: A causes B causes C causes D, and so forth. In this view, the chain of events can be traced back directly to the molecular source of the problem. Because biomedicine's goal is to counteract the molecular problem, treatment is reduced to scientific technology, either drugs or surgery, provided by a licensed physician.

Biomedicine analyzes every disease this way. For example, it is well known that the risk of heart disease is associated with high serum cholesterol. Due to biomedicine's "A causes B" mentality, it's assumed that the cholesterol molecule is the sole cause, the break in the chain, so to speak. To reduce the risk of heart disease then, doctors prescribe drugs that inhibit the body's production of cholesterol. From this perspective, our emotions, the food we eat, how much we exercise, and where we live are overlooked, as are the body's tightly interlocking networks of serial processes that metabolize serum cholesterol. The former are overlooked because they don't address the molecular cause of the problem; the latter, because linear thinking can't handle serial processes.

In this linear production model in which sickness → drugs + surgery → cure, the physician is the healer and is responsible for producing health. Health, implicitly, is something the doctor produces because he is the sole proprietor of the scientific knowledge needed to diagnose and treat disease. The patient is perceived as a passive recipient of the doctor's care. Any notion of enough is moot because linear thinking encourages us to believe that technology—if not this generation's, the next—can control nature, defeat death and disability, and delay aging.

In the United States, the ascendancy of biomedicine occurred between 1850 and 1930 and was guided by medical doctors. Paul Starr refers to this period as "medicine's civil war and reconstruction."[2] It was a particularly volatile period of creativity in U.S. history. Corporations were granted legal status; mining, manufacturing and railroads created new concentrations of wealth; public education became compulsory; and the population expanded westward. Although initiated earlier and completed later, the center of economic and social life continued its long, slow shift from the family to the corporation.

During this eighty-year period, medical doctors consolidated their power and privilege through educational credentialing and the enactment of licensing laws, and care of the sick became a professional responsibility rather than a woman's domestic chore. By claiming their training was scientific and by making licensure dependent on attending medical school, physicians were singularly successful in garnering the knowledge power. As a result, the other sects of healers—homeopaths, naturopaths, Christian Science practitioners, midwifes, and all other types of practitioners who had other training but did not qualify for licensure—found themselves outside health care's boundaries. By the 1950s, health insurance regulations had guaranteed the profession's market-power, thereby finalizing the medical profession's monopoly over potential competitors.

Due to decades of innovation, nineteenth-century practitioners would scarcely recognize today's practice of biomedicine, or health care. Such things as corporate management, organ transplants, cosmetic surgery, genetic engineering, nursing homes, and designer drugs have remodeled health care. However, ideas about healer, patient, cause, and remedy have basically remained the same.

As much as market forces and the scientific revolution determined the outcome of medicine's civil war and reconstruction, health care's organizing force still emanates from the modern worldview. Modernity's values—materialism, reductionism, and determinism—are so integral to health care as to be unquestioned, yet these values generate much of what we resent: the engineering model of the body, the lack of caring, and the commodification of health. Reducing the patient to biochemical molecules, modernity fosters the perception that nature can be controlled and presents the patient as an isolated, self-contained physical body, separate from the rest of the population, separate from the environment, and separate from the divine.

HEALTH IS THE CAPACITY TO WORK

Although beliefs about the objectivity of science allow health care to be perceived as neutral and free of social influences, health defined as the capacity to work is a stark reminder that neither the definition of health nor health care is objective. Both are shaped as much by the era's political and economic imperatives as by its science.

That health is the capacity to work was first promulgated by the Rockefeller Foundation in the early years of the twentieth century and is a variation on biomedicine's definition of health. Historically, the definition coincides with U.S. imperialism. Ironically, it also coincides with the European inception of universal health benefits.

Frederick T. Gates, the chief lieutenant for John D. Rockefeller Sr.'s financial empire and philanthropies, understood the political consequences of biomedicine's singular concern with disease as germ-caused. "In brief, Gates embraced scientific medicine as a force that would: 1) help unify and integrate the emerging industrial society with technical values and culture, and 2) legitimize capitalism by diverting attention from structural and environmental causes of disease."[3] To achieve its own interests, the Rockefeller Foundation endowed select medical schools committed to scientific and technological approaches to health.

Late in the nineteenth century, when U.S. industrialists were looking to the rural South and to undeveloped countries for new resources, markets, and investment opportunities, biomedicine was enjoying high public confidence. For the first time, death rates from infectious disease—then the leading cause of death—were dropping. Medical science had identified most of the microbes that caused cholera, tuberculosis, yellow fever, and other infectious diseases. Between the use of vaccines and the implementation of public health measures—such as clean drinking water, sewage systems, and the clearing of slums—biomedicine took credit for noticeably reducing the severity and frequency of infectious diseases. Within this nexus, the Rockefeller Foundation championed the formation of local public health departments staffed by full-time public health officers and provided the first major funding for schools of public health in the United States and overseas.

Expecting the application of medical technology to increase corporate profits, the foundation's interest in public health was as much opportunistic as altruistic. On one hand, infectious disease would no longer rob workers of productivity, nor would business be lost to infectious epidemics. On the other, biomedicine was a powerful social influence and a soft sell. By preventing and treating infectious diseases, biomedicine readily induced native populations to adopt American values and its industrial way of life, while also assuring U.S. access to these new markets.[4]

The Rockefeller definition generates the same linear production model as biomedicine's. However, its outcome is specific and easy to measure: sickness $\rightarrow$ drugs + surgery $\rightarrow$ productivity. Improvements in health are measured by quantitative increases in worker productivity.

Defining health as the ability to do productive work tacitly explains why health benefits are tied to employment. When health is defined as the capacity to work, many people are excluded. Also, the Rockefeller definition implies that health care's purpose is commercial. It is neither effective nor efficient to spend resources on those who are too young, too old, too infirm, too feeble-minded, too uncooperative, too uneducated, or too disabled to be economically productive.

HEALTH IS A STATE OF COMPLETE PHYSICAL, MENTAL, AND SOCIAL WELL BEING, NOT JUST THE ABSENCE OF DISEASE

In 1948, twenty-six nations ratified the charter for the World Health Organization (WHO). An agency of the United Nations, WHO's purpose was to act as the directing and coordinating authority on international health. Framers of the WHO charter described health as "a state of complete physical, mental, and social well-being and not merely the absence of disease or infirmity."[5] Forty years later, the United Nation's International Covenant on Economic, Social, and Cultural Rights recognized "the *right* [italics added] of everyone to the enjoyment of the highest attainable standard of physical and mental health."[6] The United States has yet to ratify this covenant.

The origin of the WHO definition was the conviction that world peace lay in the improvement of health, physically, mentally, and socially. On one hand, war causes a violent loss of life and limb, infectious diseases follow military movement, and epidemics break out in refugee populations displaced by war. On the other hand, war is easily provoked in societies destabilized by pollution and poverty with their attendant overcrowding, poor sanitation, malnutrition, and feelings of powerlessness and social exclusion. Seeing both sides of the coin, so to speak, the framers believed that uprooting the vectors of disease would stabilize society; obversely, stabilizing society would uproot the vectors of disease.

Emerging during U.S. optimism following World War II, the WHO definition of health is as expansive as it is optimistic. The war had just been successfully fought. Employers had agreed to continue their wartime wage policy of paying for workers' health benefits. Science was advancing at a phenomenal pace, and the benefits of technology seemed endless.

Postwar advances in biochemistry were changing the practice of medicine. For the first time, the body was understood at the subcellular level. The discovery of life-saving sophisticated laboratory tests and the development of wonder drugs—antibiotics, chemotherapy, and psychotropics—strengthened the notion that technology could cure disease.

The effect of the WHO definition of health was additive, not transformative. Like blowing air into a balloon, the WHO definition fostered the economic growth of biomedicine. On one hand, physicians continued to expand their authority through the marriage of third-party reimbursement and technology. The development of behavior-controlling drugs abetted the expansion of medical authority into domains that once belonged to religious and legal authorities. Behavioral problems such as madness, alcoholism, and hyperactivity were given a medical diagnosis and a code for third-party reimbursement. Likewise, social problems such as teen pregnancies, suicides, substance abuse, violence, and other social problems were also medicalized.

On the other hand, the public, too, began to equate medical care with health. Health became conflated with perfection, and "a pill for every ill" became society's mantra. While the WHO definition addresses psychological and social well-being as aspects of health, biomedicine remains steadfast to the "germs and genes" theory of disease and modernity's linear production model. This has led to tremendous incoherence and a loss of boundaries. It is heretical to attribute symptoms to psychological, social, or spiritual causes; legitimate symptoms are adamantly attributed to biological factors. At the same time, it's in the economic best interest of providers, drug companies, purveyors of medical goods, and even medical researchers to interpret health in the broadest terms possible.

The effect is a deleterious loss of financial and moral boundaries. Daniel Callahan, a well-known bioethicist, succinctly describes the consequences of a definition of health that has no boundaries.

The consequences of this definition, or at least of the ambitious spirit which it represents, can be seen all around us. Health so defined can encompass every human state. This bottomless conceptual pit makes it impossible in any practical way to specify the limits of the health enterprise, that is, to distinguish what is a political, or ethical, or cultural problem from what is a "health" problem. It has even permeated our everyday speech: how many of us designate any political or cultural movement or any person we do not like as "sick?" The ground is thus laid for a limitless economic burden on society. If anything and everything from the state of prisons, the schools, and the economy to anxieties invoked by life can be called a "health problem," there is no end to the resources that can be expanded in the name of medicine to cope with these unpleasantries.[7]

Physicians are also affected by the moral-boundary loss, for they are tacitly held accountable for outcomes way beyond their capabilities. Being held accountable for outcomes beyond one's control makes effectiveness meaningless, because systems theory posits that the product can't be any better than the system that produces it. However, if the patient isn't cured—and biomedicine's implicit promise of cure is deeply embedded in the American psyche—then physicians and patients tend to blame each other. Neither can see that effectiveness is a systems issue, and the social norm of ferreting out the poor performer reinforces this blindness.

From a systems perspective, making physicians responsible for health tacitly conceals others' responsibilities. For example, more fatal heart attacks occur at 9:00 A.M. on Monday mornings than at any other time, and a 1 percent rise in unemployment leads to a 5.6 percent increase in death from heart attack and a 3.1 percent increase in death from stroke.[8] These are social ills, which biomedicine cares for after the biological damage has occurred. Unfortunately, this molecular chain of events is so taken for granted, so ingrained in our social structure, that the incoherence of downstream medical treatment is seldom noticed.

Basically, the WHO definition of health simply unbounded the concept of health to a state of perfection while maintaining biomedicine's concepts of healer, patient, and remedy. Its net effect was a deleterious loss of financial and moral boundaries. The loss of financial and moral boundaries contributes to health care's dysfunction, making efficiency untenable and effectiveness impossible to measure. The loss of boundaries also conceals those with upstream responsibilities, conceals the effect third-party payers have on health, and eclipses the patient's responsibilities toward his or her own health.

"WELLNESS MEANS ENGAGING IN ATTITUDES AND BEHAVIORS THAT ENHANCE THE QUALITY OF LIFE AND MAXIMIZE PERSONAL POTENTIAL"[9]

The mind/body connection is the basis for the variety of definitions that have to do with a relatively new way of thinking about health. *Wellness, prevention, holistic health,* and *optimal wellness* are terms used to describe the belief that health is more than the "five d's"—disease, death, discomfort, disability, and dissatisfaction.

Wellness does not have one standard definition; however, the various definitions have two things in common. One is the concept that health is a positive condition, not a negative physical event. The second is that health is comprised of interrelated components. Physical, mental, emotional, social, and spiritual components are always included in the definition of wellness, and intellectual, occupational, and/or environmental components are sometimes included. The interrelated components are dynamic, which means that they tend to go up or down together. For example, people who are sick tend to be emotionally fragile and socially withdrawn; an unhappy marriage, substance abuse, and high blood pressure are often found together.

Wellness ideas came into vogue in the 1970s with the convergence of a number of factors. Chronic disease had noticeably replaced infectious disease as the leading cause of death. Critics were complaining about health care's ineffectiveness, and business, which was complaining about health care costs, saw wellness programs as an inexpensive way to keep workers healthy. The counterculture's 1960s slogan, Power to the people, was gentrified. Its more respectable values of personal autonomy and consumer rights encouraged patients to abandon the paternalistic doctor-patient relationship in favor of taking a more active role in their own care.

Adding to the ferment, new scientific data showed that the mind and body are integrated. Discoveries in the areas of immunology, neurology, and endocrinology demonstrated that thoughts and feelings—particularly those associated with stress and alienation—have physiological consequences. The longer the damaging emotions stay turned on, like an engine running too hot, the more likely the body will break down into a variety of stress-related diseases, such as heart disease, cancer, and autoimmune disorders.

At the same time, other research had begun to associate certain personal behaviors with chronic disease. For instance, cancer, heart disease, and stroke are associated with smoking, not exercising, high-fat diets, and too much alcohol; diabetes is associated with obesity and lack of exercise; and increased motor vehicle deaths are associated with driving under the influence of alcohol and not wearing seatbelts.

The wellness definition proffers new understandings regarding the cause of sickness, the sanctioned interventions, the role of the healer, and the role of the patient. The wellness definition posits that sickness is caused by physical, mental, emotional, and spiritual factors—social and environmental factors are also sometimes included—that disrupt normal physiological processes. The patient is typically someone at risk or who already has a chronic disease; however, in contrast to the biomedical model, the patient does not have to have demonstrable pathology but can be someone at risk for disease or who feels sick despite the absence of biological lesions. The treatment is attitudinal and behavioral changes. The healer is the patient, who uses the knowledge and resources of medical doctors, counselors, therapists, and so forth. These resources are used to facilitate healing, which is contrary to biomedicine's goal of cure.

Research indicates that the wellness definition's multifactorial understanding of the cause of disease more accurately explains the cause of chronic disease than does biomedicine's single-vector concept. Thus, there was hope in some circles that attention to lifestyle factors—the generic name for a catalog of physical, mental, emotional, social, and spiritual factors—would do more to prevent disease and improve the health status of Americans than would spending more money on health care per se.

In actuality, the emergence of the wellness definition placed health care policy at a crossroads. One direction, potentially transformational, meant the implementation of social policies going well beyond current public health policies, because according to the definition, the patient could be perceived as a population as well as an individual. The other, a conservative direction more consistent with biomedicine's elements, meant assuming that the risk factors associated with chronic disease are chosen by the affected persons.[10]

Obviously, the latter road was taken. All that has changed over the past thirty years is that the importance of diet, stress management, and smoking cessation have been acknowledged, and techniques such as meditation and biofeedback have found their way into biomedicine's market basket of services. Although wellness concepts have been instrumental in legitimizing and popularizing a vast array of alternative medicine modalities among the general public, biomedicine has maintained and preserved its basic elements and its linear production model, protected existing institutions, and preserved reductionistic ways of thinking about health.

Although the wellness definition did open the door to alternative health care, by focusing on individual risk factors wellness continued to reduce health to an individual concern in the traditional biomedical sense. Individuals got sick, according to the conservative perception, because they made faulty lifestyle choices. Health improvement meant developing better health habits and coping skills. If individuals couldn't do this by themselves, they could consult a therapist or a counselor; if they wanted their insurance to pay for this, they needed—at a minimum—a doctor's order.

For many individuals, this new model of health is wonderful. Its popularity is substantiated by the fact that Americans now spend more money on alternative care than they spend out-of-pocket on biomedical care. Behavior modification, bodywork, meditation, biofeedback, herbs, and other alternative modalities are effective at reducing the severity of symptoms and enhancing the body's resistance to disease, according to patients. Moreover, patients appreciated the more empowering role, being treated as active participants in their own care instead of passive recipients.

Because the conservative road was taken, coping skills and lifestyle changes are mixed blessings, for they have been coopted by biomedicine. Lifestyle risk factors tend to be perceived as diseases themselves, and individual risk factors tend to muddy the boundaries of responsibility. The problem is, the focus on individual risk factors is not always empowering. Some patients are unable or unwilling to help themselves. Some resist lifestyle changes, preferring, for instance, the ease of a cholesterol-lowering pill to the hard work of changing their eating habits. For others, as Susan Sontag noted, accepting responsibility meant accepting blame, or being scapegoated. Cancer or heart disease was something you brought on because of a bad attitude or because you did something wrong. If you died, well, you didn't fight hard enough or have enough faith in yourself to get well.[11]

Even if blame is not overt, individual risk factors tacitly make patients responsible for factors well outside their control. Wellness integrates physical, mental, emotional, social, and spiritual factors, yet our penchant for reductionistic thinking causes us to forget that these personal determinants of health do not exist independently but are deeply rooted in our economic and social relationships. Even though the wellness definition implies self-control, important societal factors that can damage or promote health are largely beyond any one patient's control.

The high incidence of heart disease, for instance, in "Coronary Death Valley," a former coal-mining region along the Appalachian Mountains, is generally attributed to individual risk factors: cigarette smoking, high-fat diets, and sedentary lifestyles. Despite the presence of closed coal mines and a depressed economic base, the proposed intervention is personal: screening for high lipid levels, hypertension, and diabetes, and encouraging healthy habits.[12] This response is typical of health care, despite the renowned Roseto study,[13] which showed that social cohesion—strong family ties and egalitarian relationships—was far more important than individual risk factors in protecting residents of Roseto, Pennsylvania, against cardiovascular mortality.

In the end, the wellness definition of health did not change the basic elements of health care. However, the wellness definition, too, has contributed to the expansion of biomedicine. Causes—that is, unhealthy behaviors and attitudes—have become diseases that can be overridden with medical technology, such as drugs like Prozac and Mevacor, and risk factors have become new product lines. Because the boundary between disease and lifestyle factors is blurred, the wellness definition of health has expanded the consumption of traditional health care's goods and services and added new ones as well. For example, heart disease "is manifest in symptoms, or in elevated serum cholesterol measurements, or in excessive consumption of fats. All are 'diseases' and represent a 'need' for health care intervention."[14]

Summing up the problems associated with the wellness definition of health, Nancy Milio states:

Such programs have made the meaning of "health promotion" not a goal but a product; not a process to engage people in finding individual and collective ways to improve health, but an attractive, saleable package to be "added on" to consumers' lives; not a means to direct health-giving resources toward vulnerable groups and communities, but rather the focusing of information resources on the relatively affluent; not a set of health-effective program strategies but an income-preserving and income-producing technique for investors.[15]

In comparison to the biomedicine, Rockefeller, and WHO definitions of health, the wellness definition (1) integrates mind, body, and spirit; (2) deepens our understanding of the causes of sickness; and (3) changes the language of outcomes from cure to healing. Despite their differences, all four definitions focus on the individual, perceiving him or her apart from other members of his or her community and separate from his or her geophysical environment.

"A HEALTHY COMMUNITY IS ONE WHERE PEOPLE ARE SAFE, FEEL SAFE, ARE WELL INFORMED, FEEL EMPOWERED TO USE THIS INFORMATION TO MAKE CHOICES, HAVE LASTING BONDS WITH ONE ANOTHER, AND HAVE A SENSE OF MEANING IN THEIR LIVES"[16]

As with wellness, there is no one standard definition for community health. The perception that the health of the community and its citizens are intertwined is not new. Since the ancient Greeks, the locus of health has slowly shifted between two poles: the individual and the community. For Hippocrates, health was a social concern; since Descartes, the individual has been the locus of health. With the initiation of the WHO healthier communities movement in 1986, the pendulum appears to be reversing direction, moving back toward the community as the locus of health.

The earliest attempts to improve the health of cities and their citizens date back to Hippocrates. More contemporary endeavors go back to the German pathologist Rudolph Virchow and include the British public health movement of the early 1800s and the Progressive movement in the United States in the early 1900s.

Then, as today, the shift toward a population locus of health is fostered by two acknowledgments regarding health. First, the capacity of the health care system to substantially improve the health of a population is inherently limited. Second, the health of the individual and the political, environmental, and economic health of the community are mutually reinforcing.

The reciprocal link between economic and political health and physical health has been understood since the early industrial revolution. Both Edwin Chadwick, a British bureaucrat and social reformer, and Virchow pushed for public health measures, convinced that ameliorating wretched living and working conditions would do more to improve the community's health than biomedicine ever could do by treating the sick one at a time. Both understood that poverty and pollution were not just vectors for personal illness but that personal health and political health are intertwined and the absence of either one is costly to taxpayers.

An enormous amount of contemporary data show that the relationship between a country's economic growth and the physical health of its citizens is reciprocal. It's an association that generally begins in utero, but the economic effects are usually noticed in adulthood. In other words, healthy children tend to grow up to be productive citizens, whereas unhealthy children are costly to society. The data show that the societal conditions children experience in utero and during early childhood not only influence their learning abilities and behaviors and the size and strength of the future adult but also establish much of the risk for chronic diseases in adult life.

Briefly, a population definition of health represents a radical shift in answers to the elemental questions. First, the community is the patient, and the traditional patient becomes one self in a larger whole. Second, health is defined as a capacity or a resource rather than a condition.[17] Third, there are five major categories (shown in Figure 3.1) that determine the health of a population.[18] In other words, the production of the health of a population is complex, involving more than biological factors. Finally, as 80 percent of the determinants of health fall outside health care's control, physicians are not solely responsible for the production of health, and the majority of remedies are corporate and political policies that affect the social and geophysical environments.

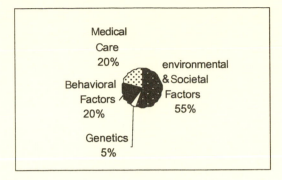

Figure 3.1 Distribution of Determinants of Health
Source: Tarlow, A. R., & St. Peter, R. F. (2000). Introduction. In A. R. Tarlow & R. F.
St. Peter (Eds.), *The Society and Population Reader: A State and Community Perspective*
(Vol. 2). New York: New Press, pp. x–xi.

Essentially, a population definition of health makes health care one system among many that affect health—not *the* system responsible for the
production of health. Accordingly, health care's boundaries are redefined,
and responsibilities are adjusted. The population's health is less the
province of health care per se and more the responsibility of the leadership of public, private and nonprofit sectors whose policies have a step-
down effect, shaping social institutions that in turn influence personal
relationships.

The remedies, or care, are policies, for interventions are aimed at environmental, economic, and social conditions that eventually damage personal physiology. According to our Canadian neighbors, the outcome then
extends beyond the health status of a single individual or a covered group
and "includes a sustainable and integrated health system, increased
national growth and productivity, and strengthened social cohesion and
citizen engagement."[19]

Although a population definition of health entails drawing new boundaries for health care, it is too early to forecast where health care's responsibilities end and the responsibilities of other institutions begin. Moreover,
it's too early to say who will assume responsibility for the coordination
and development of policies and the network of programs needed to promote the health of the whole. The healthier communities movement calls
for the formation of partnerships among the community's private, public,
and nonprofit sectors and envisions individual citizens finding new ways
to reestablish social ties, becoming more trusting and trustworthy of one
another.

CONFLICTS AND CONFUSION

Americans do not see the same health care system; different stakeholders see different systems. Throughout the United States, small groups of business leaders, insurance executives, policy analysts, researchers, and medical leaders are involved in separate conversations about how to make health care more effective and efficient. The system each one sees is, most likely, a composite of his or her favorite elements.

Our five definitions of health—biomedicine, Rockefeller, WHO, wellness, and the community—are both causes and symptoms of health care's turmoil. They are compared in Table 3.1. The biomedical definition of health informs the core elements of the U.S. health care system. That is, health is an individual concern, sickness is caused by biological factors,

Table 3.1
Comparison of the Definitions of Health

	Biomedicine	Rockefeller	WHO	Wellness	Community
Health	Prevention and cure of disease	Ability to do productive work	Complete state of physical, mental, and social well-being	Engaging in attitudes and behaviors that enhance the quality of life and maximize personal potential	Where people are safe, well informed, feel empowered, have lasting bonds, and have a sense of meaning in their lives
Healer	Physician	Physician	Physician	Patient, physician, and other therapists	Political and corporate leadership
Patient	Person with pathology	Worker with pathology	Person with pathology	Person who is sick	Population
Remedy	Drugs and surgery	Drugs and surgery	Drugs and surgery	Behavioral and attitudinal changes	Policy changes
Outcome	Cure and prevention	Cure and prevention	Cure and prevention	Healing	Increased national productivity, social cohesion, and citizen engagement

the licensed physician is the authorized healer, and capital-intensive technology (drugs and surgery) is the sanctioned intervention; the system's purpose is to prevent and cure disease. This taken-for-granted system is tightly linked to and reinforced by third-party reimbursement.

Essentially, the wellness, WHO, and Rockefeller definitions are highly compatible with biomedicine's definition of health. All four presuppose that health is an individual concern, have created new markets, and, except for wellness, they presuppose that physicians are responsible for the production of health. Despite their compatibility, however, the roots of the conflicts regarding access to care are embedded in these definitions. For instance, the WHO definition, which implies that perfect health is a right, tacitly removes all barriers to access and is in direct opposition to the Rockefeller definition, which tacitly limits access to care by defining health as the capacity to work and implicitly tying health benefits to employment.

In contrast to the other definitions, the community definition of health is concerned with the health status of populations. Its purpose is to assure that everyone has a fair chance to be healthy, and health (which is perceived as a dynamic state, or a trajectory that includes old age, chronic conditions, and death) is attributed to five factors, one of which is health care itself. Interventions include policies and programs to alleviate the causes of disease that biomedicine can't redress—such as wages, substandard housing, toxic environments, and lack of health insurance—and that are associated with a disproportionate share of health problems among specific groups of people. Two examples already cited are the high incidence of heart disease among the residents of "Coronary Death Valley," and the increase in fatal heart attacks following job layoffs. Concomitantly, responsibility for the production of health is shared among numerous social institutions, one of which is health care.

THE POTENTIAL FOR CHANGE

The NPR/Kaiser/Kennedy School poll on health care showed that Americans are leery of health care reform,[20] and rightfully so, if more disappointments like managed care are what lies ahead. However, managed care was not reform. In systems terms, managed care merely tinkered with reimbursement methods, and tinkering, or piecemeal reform as it's usually called, makes things worse. The fact that we spend 14 percent of the GDP on a health care system that contributes about 20 percent to the health status of Americans and that the health status of Americans ranks thirty-seventh in the world is clearly indicative of a dysfunctional system. Unfortunately, nothing short of systemic improvement will fix health care's access, cost, and quality problems.

Among the many things our inquiry thus far has revealed, two items stand out. First, our health care system is without financial and moral boundaries, and second, Americans largely assume that health care can defeat death and conquer disease.

The blunt reality is that health as a state of complete physical, mental, and social well-being is merely an ideal. Disease per se can never be conquered. The British epidemiologist Thomas McKeown was the first to show that types of sickness follow historical periods.[21] Diseases of deficiencies—that is, diseases caused by parasites and malnutrition—are endemic to hunter-gatherers, infectious diseases are associated with widespread migration and rapid population growth, and chronic diseases are associated with health-damaging societal factors and environmental toxins, themselves seemingly endemic to postindustrial life.

As Mervyn Susser, Kim Hooper, and Judith Richman put it, "the entire biological, social, and cultural history of a society impinges upon the present; genes, cultural and social institutions all persist, and all change, evolve, and adapt. These forces operate through Darwinian evolution and ecological adaptation and, with greater immediacy, through economic, social, and political history."[22] Disease can't be conquered—despite the promises of medical science. In an ever-changing world, each era and each society will have its own burden of sickness formed from the unavoidable failure of the human organism to adapt to social and environmental threats.

Health, then, seems to be a trajectory between birth and death that includes states of acute disease, chronic disease, and life-threatening conditions. Contrary to the implications of the biomedicine and WHO definitions, aging, sickness, and death are a natural part of the human condition. The potential for health care reform lies in directly acknowledging that we need a new definition of health.

TURNING OFF OUR AUTOMATIC PILOT

While most of us will not take part personally in the political conversations that affect the nation's health, health is still a personal concern. How we feel about our bodies, what kind of health care we seek, and when we seek it are all determined by our beliefs about health and disease. Most of us have never asked ourselves, What is health? Is it youth, beauty, longevity, productivity, happiness, something else? Is health a process, perfection, a steady state? What health problems do I depend upon my physician to treat? How important to me is the health of people I do not know or who are different from me?

These are significant questions. Essentially, society's answers to them are the thought from which health care is formed. Like other things we take for granted, most Americans seldom consider the deep beliefs that determine their decisions about health and health care. Instead, the importance placed on health, decisions about personal health habits and when to use health care, and the care of other people are generally made automatically, influenced more by Madison Avenue than by a close examination of one's own thinking.

Unfortunately, this automatic pilot assures the turmoil of the status quo. Unexamined choices preserve the existing health care system, and even seemingly free and personal choices—when made without consciously connecting them to our deep beliefs—are in actuality dictated by the modern habit of reducing health to biological pathology. This is clearly seen in the present assumptions about menopause. Prior to the 1960s, menopause was considered a natural part of aging. Once pharmaceutical companies began selling estrogen in tablet form, however, the meaning changed. Doctors and women typically thought of menopause as a medical problem to be treated with estrogen replacement therapy.

Moreover, automatic pilot can take people where they don't want to go. For example, a seventy-eight-year-old woman with metastatic ovarian cancer claimed that had she been told all of the risks, she would not have consented to the extensive surgery her doctor recommended, which she felt had destroyed what quality of life she had left. In her condition, had she thought deeply about it, health had nothing to do with longevity and everything to do with living to the fullest extent possible, although her days were numbered.

From a personal perspective, patients who don't act automatically but who have inquired into their beliefs about health and health care typically know their rights and health care's limitations. They are well informed, cogently follow their doctors' orders, and do what they can to help themselves. While they do not expect health care to give them perfect health, they do not accept inadequate care, either.

By definition, automatic pilot locks people into the narrow range of permissible choices. Automatic pilot generally locks health care reformers, who are seeking efficiency, into building better technology and making more rules about which patients can use the technology. In contrast, being aware of our thinking frees us to act according to a direct perception of the world around us.

Paradoxically, from a large-systems perspective, acting according to a direct perception of the world and automatic actions can lead to a large system's change. Over time, automatic actions tend to amplify the flaws inherent in the status quo, such as the split between the delivery and financing of health care. Things are made worse instead of better; eventually, the system becomes unstable. For instance, attempts to make health care more efficient by ratcheting down reimbursement mechanisms have simply driven up the number of Americans who don't have health insurance, can't afford health insurance, or, if they have insurance, can't afford the out-of-pocket costs.

In contrast, even though single individuals rarely influence policy or even have much say about the type of insurance their employer purchases, providers and health plans are now interested in alternative care because the public spends as much of its own money on alternative medicine as it spends on traditional health care. Health care has noticed! While it is too early to tell whether alternative care will actually change health care, the point is that the accrual of small but conscious decisions can have a positive influence on a large system's behavior.

Very few of us have the authority to change the delivery or financing of health care, so we tend to think that one individual can't do very much to make a difference. But everything that happens is built upon individual actions. Each person's actions do matter; health care does change when a critical mass of people makes the same choice.

True reform, means that our thoughts are more coherent. Because our actions are guided by our definition of health, if we hope to have a health care system that is more effective, efficient, and fair than the one we have now, we need a definition of health that can re-form health care into a more coherent whole. This means that we have deeply examined our thinking about the meaning of health, the purpose of health care, what it means to care for one another, and what is best for the health of the whole. The answers to these questions are important guides for redrawing health care's boundaries.

QUESTIONS FOR THE READER

Below is a set of questions designed to help you identify your answers to the question, What is health? The way to answer these questions is not to say yes or no. Instead, identify what each question evokes that is important to you. This means reviewing your experiences and identifying the ethical and logical arguments—as well as the facts—you use in forming your response. It also includes noticing what physical and emotional sensations these questions evoke in you.

As a result of this activity, you will gain a clearer understanding of what you desire, and you will start to see the interrelationship among the four structural elements that comprise any health care system. These two views are essential to any kind of public conversation regarding health care reform.

QUESTIONS FOR THE READER

1. What is your definition of health? Which of the five definitions of health is most similar to your own? Why? What experiences and beliefs have helped form your views?

2. Which definition do you suppose influences the way your doctor practices medicine?

3. Which definition do you suppose your health plan is based on?

4. Is health synonymous with economic productivity? Should health insurance be tied to employment?

5. Are you healthy if you have a chronic disease, are old, or have a disability? Do you expect health care to cure you, or to care for you?

6. How much of your health is dependent upon your habits and attitudes? Do your actions affect the health of others? Do the actions of others affect your health?

7. How much of your health is dependent on an adequate income, living in a safe environment, and having a voice in decisions that affect your life? If your neighbors have more or less of these, does this affect your health?

8. How much of your health is dependent on having access to a physician in whom you have confidence, access to high-quality medical facilities, and access to health insurance?

9. Suppose you or a family member is so severely injured that the body can't breathe, eat, fight infections, or regulate itself without technology. Is it health to sustain a mind that has no body? Or to sustain a body that has no mind?

10. How much of your health is dependent upon your relationships—with your family, your friends, your community, the environment, with God?

11. If we are neither cured when we are chronically ill nor able to afford all the care we need when we are old or disabled, what is the role of health care in which so much has been invested?

12. Return to your own definition of health. On what criteria did you base your definition? Who is included and who benefits? Who does your definition exclude? Make a table of your definition's structural elements.

CHAPTER 4

What Is Care?

To cure rarely, to relieve suffering often, to comfort always.

Anonymous

The word *care* has multiple meanings. One meaning is ethical, suggesting compassion, solicitude, or devotion toward the sick. Another meaning is supervisory, implying to be in charge of or responsible for some person or object. Lastly, care denotes forms of interventions or remedies used in the production of health. All three meanings pertain to our inquiry.

Because human beings and their systems are mutually enfolded, our inquiry into the question What is care? is an exploration into the thoughts that inform both the quality of human relationships and the resources used in the production of health. Of course, this presupposes that we know what health is.

When we think of the word *care*, the cliché "tender, loving care" often comes to mind. Generally speaking, care is a synonym for quality, because the term tacitly refers to the remedy and the healer's skills.

In systems language, our inquiry What is care? explores the types of resources, or inputs, used in the production of health. At this level, we are examining primarily the effectiveness of remedy. However, because health insurance pays for care, we are also looking at the influence of health insurance. This is more than asking whether are we treating the right patient with the right remedy, that is, addressing pinpoint-specific quality issues; we are actually inquiring into the health care system's capacity, its ability to be effective.

Using Flood's language, when we ask What is care? we are asking whether the healer and the remedy produce what the system purports to produce, and if not, why not. Are the remedies wrong, are the relationships wrong, or is our definition of health wrong? This kind of mini–check and balance because a coherent health care system means that our definition of health is in alignment with our ideas regarding the cause of sickness, the healer, the patient, and the remedy.

THE RELATIONSHIP BETWEEN HEALTH INSURANCE AND CARE

Anthropologists posit two opposing ways societies care for their sick. In one, the sick person is either abandoned or leaves the group until recovery or death ensues. In the other, the sick person is cared for by others, fed, and protected until he or she can care for him- or herself.

Americans fit somewhere in between. Not everyone has access to health *care*. Access largely depends upon whether one has health insurance, and access to health insurance is largely dependent upon employment. The two exceptions are the elderly, who have Medicare, and the very poor, who have Medicaid. Unfortunately, not every American with a health problem is included in the patient stakeholder group; the U.S. health care system generally excludes those without insurance.

Though largely ignored as a determinant of health care's effectiveness, health insurance directly and indirectly contributes to the quality of the health of individuals and the population. First, access to care largely depends upon health insurance. For example, it's well known that the health status of people without insurance is generally poorer. The uninsured are less likely to receive preventive care or routine care for chronic conditions, are more likely to be hospitalized for conditions that could have been avoided with timely outpatient intervention, and have a higher in-hospital death rate. Moreover, the uninsured tend to die younger.

Second, health insurance significantly influences the configuration of the U.S. health care system. A powerful force, health insurance serves to maintain biomedicine's monopoly and to protect it against potential competition from other types of healers and their remedies. In addition, most forms of health insurance enable providers and purveyors to escalate their fees ceaselessly.

SEEING THE CURRENT INCOHERENCE

Americans are tacitly aware of health care's incoherence, although they wouldn't articulate the cause as a misalignment between biomedical elements and the WHO product (see Figure 4.1). In everyday language, it's generally spoken of as exorbitant costs or a wish to be cared for as a whole person.

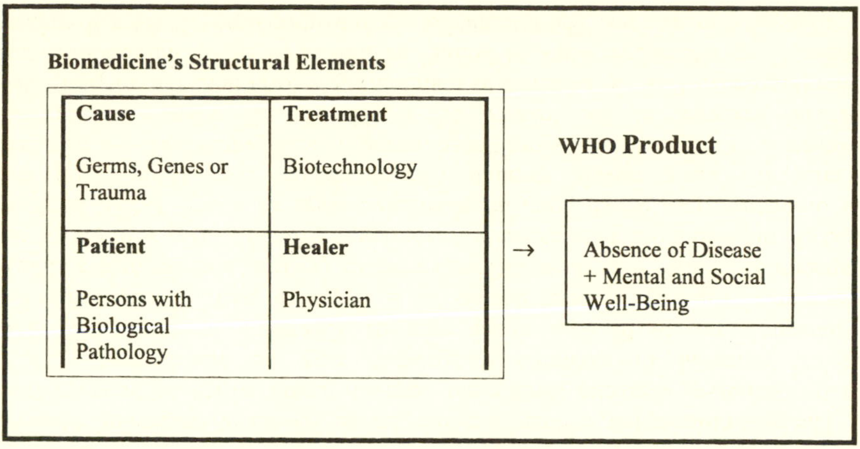

Biomedicine's Structural Elements

Cause	Treatment		WHO Product
Germs, Genes or Trauma	Biotechnology		
Patient	**Healer**	→	Absence of Disease + Mental and Social Well-Being
Persons with Biological Pathology	Physician		

Figure 4.1 The Current Health Care System: Elements ≠ Product

To illustrate, biomedicine is highly effective for those who require sophisticated surgical and medical interventions and for those who require high-tech monitoring. Certainly, organ transplantation, artificial joints, kidney dialysis, powerful antibiotics, and home glucose-monitoring tests have directly contributed to a longer and more comfortable life for many people. However, the optimism and expansiveness are now a mixed blessing. Having reduced menopause, aging, and even death—natural stops along the trajectory of life—to metabolic processes, the idea of perfection contributes to some very confused relationships.

In the biomedical model, the body is perceived as an inert object, and the mind is separate from the body. Accordingly, the patient is *acontextual*, an independent entity, a cosmos unto itself. Consequently, environmental and psychosocial factors—such as polluted water, stressful jobs, racial and economic marginalization, anger, guilt, and loneliness, all known to affect the biochemistry of the mind/body ensemble—are either ignored or conveniently overridden by biotechnology.

As Howard F. Stein says, "Problems are looked for, sought out, located, defined, identified, isolated, and treated inside the human body."[1] Even psychiatry treats the mind/body ensemble as an object. Depression, learning disabilities, and other disturbances in mood and cognition are viewed as caused by abnormalities of the brain's biochemistry and are cured by mind-altering pharmaceuticals. Unfortunately, this so-called objectivity contributes to the patient's alienation from him- or herself and fosters unrealistic expectations that health care's armamentarium of biotechnology can return the body to its preinjured state.

This objectivity also makes biomedicine largely blind to the emotional and financial toll chronic and life-threatening sickness take on the patients' and their family's resources. For patients and their families, sickness is more than a biological event. Drugs and surgery alone are incapable of ameliorating suffering.

Trapped in the reductionistic methodology of health care, physicians often find themselves caring for the patient's broken body part without ever comforting the mind and spirit. This is not because physicians are heartless or thoughtless; it is because the health care system mirrors our perception of the body. In keeping with modernity's materialistic exemplars, both are perceived as if they were mechanical clocks. In the name of efficiency, bureaucratic mechanisms tightly ration the provider's time and resources.

This is as hard on providers as it is on patients. The doctor-patient relationship is reduced to double-entry accounting and cost effectiveness ratios. When an eight-minute office visit is the standard, it is efficient—though not always effective—to focus on objective laboratory data and quickly fix the broken part.

Medical training is based on materialistic, reductionistic exemplars, and physicians are taught to be objective. The material view of health causes providers to be preoccupied with scientific competency, which means providing a biologically accurate diagnosis and technically competent treatment. Cure or relief of symptoms is the output of a competent physician. Thus, if a woman's broken arm bone knits, the physician is not concerned that the patient can't braid her hair or hoe her garden, or that her medical bill will leave her bankrupt. Believing that he or she has successfully fulfilled his or her obligation, the physician is unaware that these subjective losses can cause the patient to suffer or question the physician's competency.

Furthermore, there is a definite limit to health care's effectiveness in treating one patient at a time with medical technology. To illustrate, black males who live in Washington, D.C., the Oglala Sioux, and the homeless have a life expectancy of between fifty-five and fifty-nine years, lower than that of many people living in third world countries.[2] Essentially, advances in medical technology account for an estimated 25 percent of increases in longevity,[3] while the remaining 75 percent is due to improvements in nutrition, housing, sanitation, occupational safety, and lifestyle.

Our thoughts that inform the current health care system are incoherent. In short, the current health care system can never be effective because, as we now conceive it, health care is fashioned from biomedicine's understanding of healer, patient, remedy, and cause of sickness. However, our definition of health is the WHO definition, which implies that health is a state of perfection. This taken-for-granted incoherence is tightly linked to and reinforced by third-party reimbursement and modernity's scientific concepts.

A POSTMODERN UNDERSTANDING OF HEALTH
AND CARE

Sustained inquiry takes us to new levels of understanding. That is its purpose. Much as learning a foreign language provides insight into the construction of one's native language, seeing the multiple definition of health provides us with a clearer understanding of each definition's limitations. Having moved to new levels of understanding, we can say our thought is freed from the mooring of status quo thinking, or that we are freed from the default of automatic pilot.

In fact, when our understanding of health is loosened from its moorings of modern, linear thinking, our ideas about care shift as well. To continue our inquiry into What is care? is to understand even more about the organization of our current health care system, because this question illuminates the concepts that inform our percepts of cause, remedy, and healer. It is in this illumination that new and more coherent ways for improving health care's effectiveness are revealed.

In our emerging understanding of health, three interrelated principles are becoming clear. First, the WHO notion of perfect health is merely an ideal. We now know that health is more a dynamic than a steady state, and we know that health is as much a population concern as it is an individual concern. In fact, if we define health as a capacity instead of as a steady state or an ideal of perfection, it seems rational to think of health as a range of population and individual needs—prevention and acute, chronic, and life-threatening—that health care is popularly expected to redress.

The second emerging principle is that a single biological vector seldom causes sickness, any more than exposure to a cold virus guarantees a cold. Instead, sickness is usually the result of multiple causes accumulated under the right circumstances. From this it follows that the body does not exist as an independent entity. Health can't be controlled with the precision of a simple chemical reaction in an Ehrlemeyer flask. Rather, human beings are part of a larger whole; health and sickness depend upon the context of people's lives.

Human life is one of the most tightly coupled systems in the universe. We are linked to our external world through our five senses. Our eyes, ears, nose, mouth, and skin are portals, so to speak, bringing the external environment to the physical self. The material world is incorporated into our physical being through the food and water we eat and drink and the air we breathe. Social and personal encounters likewise affect us because they too are incorporated into our physiology. Simply speaking, our encounters with the external world trigger an internal stream of biological events that our computerlike mind ultimately reduces to one decision: Are we safe, or are we in danger? In a split second, the mind translates a cascade of neural, endocrine, and immune reactions into emotions. Despite the claim that our decisions are logical and rational, in truth, our decisions are determined by a feeling: pleasure or pain.

The goal of these very basic regulatory mechanisms is survival, and for the most part they operate outside our awareness. Generally, we are only aware of these mechanisms when the body talks back. That is, after compensatory mechanisms have been turned on long enough to become pathology. In other words, we typically feel the headache and then notice the clenched jaw; or we experience the chest pain and then discover our high cortisol, catecholamine, and cholesterol levels.

Around 1970, scientists began identifying what are called *determinants of health.* These are factors from the world outside the body that affect the body's metabolic mechanisms. The Canadian Health Network lists eleven significant factors: income and social status, social support networks, employment and working conditions, education, physical environments, genetics, personal health habits and coping skills, healthy child development, health services, gender, and culture.[4]

Dynamic and interrelated, the determinants of health tend to go up and down together, forming the confluence of causes, conditions, and circumstances that determine health. The more positive factors people have in their lives, generally, the healthier they are. To put it another way, sickness occurs when there is enough negative accumulation to damage the body's biological pathways.

To illustrate, the genes BRCA1 and BRCA2, environmental pollutants, estrogen replacement therapy, diet, cigarette smoking, and childlessness are all risk factors associated with breast cancer. Although scientists vigorously debate whether one factor is more lethal than others, how much and how long a factor needs to be present to cause damage, and whether some combinations are more deadly than others, no one claims that breast cancer is attributable to one lethal factor.

The determinants of health lead to the third emerging principle, that health is also a population concern. Briefly, population health refers to the health status of a whole, of a group of people who share a common geography, class, race, age, or gender. In other words, they tend to have the same determinants of health in common. This is why the health status of the individual largely mirrors that of his or her neighbors. For instance, the highest rates of death from heart disease are not randomly scattered throughout the United States but occur largely in one place known as the "Coronary Death Valley," an area that includes most of the part of Appalachia characterized by unemployment, isolation, and poor health habits.

From a population perspective (shown in Figure 3.3), social and environmental factors are at least twice as important to the production of health as medical care is. This means that it's neither effective nor efficient to intervene with medical technology after the stress of poverty, troublesome relationships, or breathing polluted air manifests itself as heart dis-

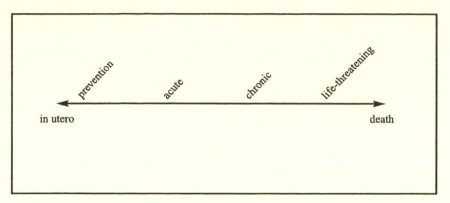

Figure 4.2 Continuum of States

ease, domestic violence, or asthma. Intervening after the problem becomes molecular pathology is like closing the barn door after the horse has escaped. Such behavior is as inefficient and ineffective as treating cholera victims—one at a time—with rehydration therapy and intravenous antibiotics instead of providing the community with clean water and sanitation.

A postmodern understanding of health and care illuminates important reasons why the current, linear production model sickness → drugs + surgery → cure is not effective. From the three principles, it follows that the production of health is far more complicated than access to medical care. Medical care represents roughly 20 percent of the determinants of health, another 25 percent belong to the patient, and social and environmental factors represent roughly another 55 percent.

Moreover, if we define health as a capacity, instead of as a steady state or an ideal of perfection, then it follows that in order for care to be effective, a range of remedies is needed to match a continuum of needs: prevention and acute, chronic, and life-threatening needs (see Figure 4.2). These needs are associated with the terms *health* and *care*.

NO CLEAR PURPOSE

We expect good health from our health care system. We tell one another that we have the best health care system in the world. As we've noted, however, Americans in fact have the most expensive health care system in the world, with less coverage, lower life expectancy, and higher infant mortality rates than nations with universal health coverage. Paying top-end prices, one expects a high-quality product. The data indicate the public isn't getting what it is paying for.

Effectiveness refers to doing the right thing. What is the right thing? Because right depends upon purpose, cynics would say that health care is effective. Pointing to the data, they'd say that health care's purpose is to maximize profits and claim that the sick are simply resources to be used in the production of profits.

Even those who posit a more humane purpose disagree regarding the purpose of health care. On one side are the proponents of traditional bio-medicine who reduce care to drugs and surgery. These proponents truth-fully believe that the individual is the rightful object of care and the physician is a scientist who should concentrate on a biologically accurate diagnosis and technically competent treatment. Cure and relief of symp-toms are the output of this form of care. Simply put, it is the mechanical clock argument.

On the other side are proponents of the goldfish-bowl argument. Aware of postmodern principles, they argue that health care is one system of many affecting the health of the whole population. They understand that environmental hazards and social inequalities impact the health of the whole population and account for about 55 percent of the burden of dis-ease. They also recognize the ineffectiveness of biomedicine's efforts to reduce the treatment of chronic and life-threatening conditions to the same limited remedy—drugs and surgery—used to treat acute conditions.

Briefly, postmodern proponents see that health is a capacity associated with a range of needs. Because they distinguish among caring, curing, and healing, postmodern proponents also see multiple levels of care. These are similar to Maslow's hierarchy of needs and correspond to the five cate-gories of the determinants of health. Some levels belong solely to health care itself, some belong to the patient, and some are shared with or belong to other social systems.

We will follow these two threads of thought. Deepening our inquiry into the question What is care? should lead to insights that can re-form health care into a more effective system.

CARING, CURING, AND HEALING

Our inquiry so far shows the moral, resource, and responsibility impli-cations of care. Like the word *health*, the term *care* evokes inconsistent images in people's minds. Just as nouns create pictures in our heads, verbs have a power of their own. Their images set in motion something almost unstoppable, for meanings determine actions, yet meanings shift with the vagaries of politics and time. *Caring, curing,* and *healing* are old and com-plicated words. Used interchangeably, they form movable boundaries, making health care resemble a shell game, clouding responsibilities, and concealing what patients and populations can rightfully expect.

To cure means to restore function: The bone is set, coronary arteries are unplugged, the brain's biochemistry is balanced. Curing is not the same as healing. Their differences are apparent in their roots. The term *healing* comes from *healen,* the root of interrelated concepts: healthy, holy, whole. To cure, however, has its roots in duty, a meaning that makes cure akin to medical competence.

By calling itself health *care,* however, the images of care belong to biomedicine, even though technical competence by the provider is all that health care promises. Caring includes curing, yet it means much, much more. Care connotes comfort and compassion. Care is a reflection back to the patient of his capacities, of what he can do for himself. Care is also witnessing the patient's experience, a way of listening that entails letting the patient be sick in her own way rather than expecting her to be the doctor's idea of a good patient.

Care promotes a population's as well as the patient's good. Care is support and a removal of barriers. Thus care emphasizes moral disposition rather than moral principles and is more about responsibilities and relationships than mastery and being in control of the patient's health.

Caring fosters healing, although it would be erroneous to say caring causes healing. *To heal* means to make whole. Healing is always unique, and in the context of human life, healing is a deeply personal experience, for healing involves the restoration of integrity. Healing is the dissolution of exploitive boundaries: between mind, body, and spirit; between self and others; between humans and the biosphere. Healing is a profound sense of coherence—even if the body dies.

MASLOW'S HIERARCHY OF NEEDS

The psychologist Abraham Maslow was among the first to understand that health is dependent upon the interaction of levels of needs, or multiple determinants. The levels within Maslow's hierarchy of needs are not a linear progression, but, like the five categories of the determinants of health, they function synergistically.

1. Physiological needs. The need for food, water, oxygen, and shelter. These biological needs are basic because without them, humans would quickly die.

2. Safety needs. The need to be safe, or away from dangerous situations, violent people, and hazardous places.

3. Belonging and love needs. The need to escape loneliness and alienation, to belong, to be accepted, to give and receive love.

4. Prestige and esteem needs. The need to feel competent and respected, to have one's contributions acknowledged and appreciated.

5. Self-actualization needs. The need to be authentic, to be happy, to be engaged in meaningful activities, and to have a reverence for life.[5]

Maslow saw human beings as highly complex biological systems whose health depends upon a continuum of needs. While the five needs are interdependent, they are also graduated. In other words, we need a lot more of some things than we do of others. Maslow depicted this hierarchy as a pyramid. Those needs at the bottom of the pyramid are the things most essential to us. They are the basic physiological needs for safety and shelter, whose absence will quickly kill us. In the middle are the social interactions we depend on to know who we are. At the top of the pyramid, Maslow placed those things we need less often or less of. Some people can spend their entire life without ever needing God, yet none of us can go without oxygen for very long.

According to Maslow, the healthiest people are those for whom all five levels of needs are met. In contrast, people preoccupied with meeting basic physiological and safety needs are struggling to survive.

HEALTH CARE IS MORE THAN DRUGS AND SURGERY

We live in a time when health care's ineffectiveness is noticeable. We know the contemporary structure neither prevents causes significant to the population's health, manages chronic and life-threatening conditions adequately, nor redresses the difficult and often devastating effects sickness has on a patient's spirit and psyche and on his or her family's finances. We also live in a time of turmoil and experimentation. It stands to reason that having multiple definitions of health, we'd also have multiple ideas regarding care.

Within this turmoil, innovators are experimenting with a wide variety of interventions. These remedies range from antibiotics to social capital, from clean air to prayer. It is interesting to note that these remedies can be arranged to fit Maslow's hierarchy of needs and are consistent with the continuum of needs—prevention and acute, chronic, and life-threatening —involved in the production of health.

To a large extent, the experimentation and innovation have to do with the renewed interest in population health, the changing patterns of disease, and health care's inability to redress suffering. What is new is that care is not reduced to drugs and surgery, and human beings are not collapsed to their physical body. Instead, levels of care are emerging out of the research. Some forms of care belong solely to health care itself, some belong to the patient, and some are shared with or belong to other social systems.

Ultimately, Americans will need to ask themselves the boundary-setting questions, What forms of care belong to health care? What forms are needed to make the system more effective? Based on our personal understanding of the cause of sickness and our own definition of health, each one of us has a favorite selection of remedies we'd like our health plan to cover. These days, covered benefits are the focus of the public's attention, for they largely determine personal access to health care. However, even though population remedies seem more distant to our needs than covered benefits, our awareness should include the level of remedies that affect the population's health. Each one of us is a part of that whole.

So that we can better see the evolving continuum of remedies useful to the production of health, care is categorized, similar to Maslow's hierarchy of needs. For each category (the subjects of the next five sections), the benefits and limitations are explained.

BEHAVIORAL DETERMINANTS OF HEALTH, OR MIND/BODY MEDICINE

Norman Cousins was among the first to draw serious attention to the mind/body connection with his now-famous book *Anatomy of an Illness*. In it he describes his remarkable recovery from a painful form of arthritis by laughing himself well.[6]

Relatively new, behavioral medicine has grown with the rapidly developing field of psychoneuroimmunology (PNI), the scientific study of subtle metabolic connections among the immune, neurological, and endocrine systems. The subsequent association of chronic diseases with poor coping skills and poor personal health habits, and the rise of the consumer movement with its emphasis on informed participation in one's own care have also contributed to the evolution of behavioral care.

Behavioral therapies are designed to modify thoughts, feelings, behaviors, and cognitive skills. Generally speaking, such interventions fall into four categories: self-expression, self-regulation, behavior modification, and self-care. They help people better cope with their afflictions. Because of their diversity, these interventions are offered through a wide range of practitioners: psychologists, social workers, counselors, nurses, allied health personnel, and physicians. Despite their differences in titles and training, their common denominator is the assumption that thoughts, feelings, and cognitive skills affect health.

Self-expression therapies—such as journaling and art, dance, and music therapy—deepen people's emotional and physical integration. Because these therapies engage one or more of the senses, they encourage creativity and enable patients to become more aware of and able to describe, express, and share the stream of thoughts, feelings, and experiences that result from being sick. Exposing what's been repressed or hidden, self-expression therapies bring patients closer to the truth of their condition. Moreover, the selections and rejections that go into creating the art give patients with chronic disease, terminal illness, and intractable pain a new sense of control and a connection to a broader, deeper spectrum of meaning and value.

Self-regulation therapies—such as hypnosis, biofeedback, meditation, and stress management techniques—teach people to modulate their autonomic nervous system. Improved coping skills can reduce the frequency and discomfort of problems such as migraine headaches, irritable bowel syndrome, angina and cardiac disrhythmias, and acne and other skin problems and can aid in the maintenance of more normal blood pressure and blood sugar levels. Besides reducing the severity and frequency of physical symptoms, self-regulation therapies also speed recovery from trauma and infectious diseases and enhance the body's resistance to disease.

Self-care and behavior modification activities teach cognitive skills. Basically, behavior modification is a method of motivating people to improve their diets, stop smoking, exercise more, overcome substance abuse, and refrain from other reckless behaviors. Often modeled after Alcoholics Anonymous, behavior modification develops healthy habits that protect against disease.

In contrast, self-care refers to the strengthening of patients' abilities to manage their chronic health problems day by day. Self-care teaches the patient how to monitor and take appropriate actions, remain physically active and involved in supportive relationships, solicit information from providers regarding treatment options, and express expectations and preferences regarding functional goals for leading a satisfying, productive life.

Mind/body care is still evolving. In 1979, when Cousins published *Anatomy of an Illness*, mind/body therapies were discounted by most of the medical community. Today, due to controlled trials across a range of chronic conditions and scientific evidence offered by PNI investigations, mind/body therapies are generally acceptable to physicians—though rarely prescribed and seldom covered by health insurance.

Why don't most health plans cover behavioral care? Critics point to the lack of scientific proof that mind/body interventions can actually cure. Moreover, almost every physician has a horror story of a patient who tried to think herself well. Others know of patients whose symptoms coincided with stressful jobs and forced retirements. When the patient finally gave up herbs and stress management and sought medical care, a rapidly growing cancer or some other metabolic disaster was discovered.

The criticisms are more complicated, however. Valid clinical studies do show the effectiveness of mind/body therapies. They have been proven to aid in the recovery from the shock of a life-threatening diagnosis, reduce the severity and frequency of symptoms, lessen the side effects of treatment, improve daily functioning, help patients mobilize resources of their own, and reduce the utilization of traditional health care resources.[7]

However, the benefits are inconsistent and depend upon a variety of factors, such as the quality of mind/body interventions, their integration with other medical treatment, the type and severity of the sickness, and the patient's motivation and capacity to engage in mind/body care. In addition, mind/body care requires time, trust, and collaboration between the provider and the patient. But the thoughts, feelings, and cognitive skills are resources that belong to the patient and are outside the provider's control. Although the provider influences how the patient uses these resources, their effectiveness is far more organic than mechanistically predictable.

Unhappily, the collusion to maintain biomedicine's status quo runs deep. Having to work and be responsible on their own behalf is anathema to patients looking for quick fixes and magic bullets. And as long as physicians are paid by procedures, they have little incentive to use mind/body therapies that take up a great deal of their time.

The good news is that mind/body care is useful in the maintenance of health and in conjunction with biomedical management of chronic disease. Mind/body interventions are noninvasive and relatively low-cost. Instead of curing, they promote healing. Mind/body therapies reduce the severity and frequency of symptoms, reduce the consumption of biotechnological resources, reduce suffering, and give patients a greater sense of control over their own destiny. Patients learn to be reasonably functional instead of feeling incapacitated and powerless.

INTIMATE RELATIONSHIPS AND HEALTH

The cardiologist Dean Ornish, M.D., has done more to call attention to intimate relationships as a remedy than any other American physician. While acknowledging the power of lifestyle changes, by-pass surgery, and drugs in the management of heart disease, Ornish writes that

increasing scientific evidence from my own research and from other studies that cause me to believe that love and intimacy are among the most powerful factors in health and illness, even though these ideas are largely ignored by the medical profession.... Love and intimacy are at the root of what makes us sick and what makes us well, what causes sadness and what brings happiness, what makes us suffer and what leads to healing. If a new drug had the same impact, virtually every doctor in the country would be recommending it for their patients.[8]

Intimacy heals; in contrast, isolation damages. For example, babies kept warm, dry, and fed but isolated from the caress of human touch and voice were more likely to die than those who were talked to and played with by the staff of an orphanage. Widowers had a 40 percent greater risk of dying in the first year following their wife's death. Persons with heart disease who did not have someone to confide in were three times more likely to die early from their disease than were those who were married or had a close friend. A nine-year follow-up study of Alameda County, California residents showed that after adjusting for socioeconomic status and poor health habits, those who were least socially connected were twice as likely to die from all causes as were those with family or social ties.[9]

Relationships refer to love and belonging, a feeling of being cared for, of having someone you can count on. This emotional bond gives us permission to be changed by sickness and disability; to reweave identities, assume new roles, adjust responsibilities, and still be loved, warts and all. Relationships can't be taken like a pill. One is not a passive recipient of this form of care. Much as stamina and strength are increased with exercise, relationships—feelings of love and intimacy—are cultivated by learning to give, receive, grieve, trust, and forgive in equal measure.

When the emotional bonds between patient and caregiver are weak, mutual resentments, feelings of inadequacy, fears of losing control, and fears of being a burden and of being burdened tend to fester. Then, the teenage diabetic's blood sugar is perpetually out of control, despite—or because of—parental admonition. The cancer patient dies alone and in pain. Angry about his unraveling life, convinced he is a burden, the father's sullen anger drives his family further away.

How relationships produce health is not well understood. Some researchers believe that feeling valued fosters self-efficacy, or the confidence to think and behave in new ways. Others believe relationships buffer the damaging effects of stress, nourish a sense of hope, and foster a sense of meaning or give coherence to life. Studies show that feeling cared about and valued by others—despite altered roles and physical limitations—help the sick maintain a sense of optimism, which enhances the immune system. This may explain why women with metastatic breast cancer who belonged to a support group were likely to live twice as long as those without the benefit of psychosocial support.[10] Even beyond such health-producing metabolic effects, it's a fact that we need others to protect us and provide for us when we can't care for ourselves.

Relationships are not substitutes for biomedical care, and biomedical care is not a substitute for intimacy and protection. They are important adjuncts to each other. The chronically ill, the frail elderly, the disabled, and the dying depend on others to protect and provide for them not as mechanical objects but as feeling human beings. Having someone to count on without having to hide the true nature of your condition cultivates feelings of belonging and value, buffering the damaging effects of sickness, and the dreadfulness of death. It seems the very act of caring evokes profound changes in the physiology of both the patient and the other.

The active ingredient is the quality of the emotional bond between the patient and the caregiver. It is through these connections that we undo the delusion of separation and learn to know ourselves in a larger sense. Quoted in Ornish, John Kabat-Zinn says, "With this sense of knowing comes a kind of profound relaxation that the body responds to by restoring itself to whatever is the deepest homeostatic balance it is capable of."[11]

Some would include relationships in the mind/body category; however, they are not the same remedy. Although both have a relatively direct motivational, emotional, or neuroendocrine effect that promotes health in the face of either stress or other health hazards, the difference is that the emotional bonds of relationships operate independently of cognitive skills, coping styles, and adaptability.[12]

Like mind/body interventions, the providers' titles and training for relationship interventions vary widely. While relationships are primarily family and friends, relationship care typically includes support groups, psychotherapy, and communication skills. Generally not a covered benefit, patients must seek this care for themselves. Some notable exceptions include the federal government–sponsored Senior Companion, a companion program for isolated elderly; Ornish's cardiac rehabilitation programs; and some hospice programs.

SOCIETAL DETERMINANTS OF HEALTH

If love is the critical resource in relationships, then inclusion is the form of care in short supply regarding societal determinants of health. Inclusion refers to respect and autonomy, and is described as the power to pursue one's goals, the freedom to choose, and/or the right to make demands on other people. Societal determinants, such as income, race, education, gender, and occupation, affect a person's autonomy and what others think of him or her. More broadly, societal determinants refer to social structure— the norms, values, sanctions, privileges, and obligations—that organize social relationships. These relationships, in turn, inform social institutions, such as law and health care. Societal determinants are our collective way of saying who is in and who is out.

The link between societal determinants and sickness is clear. It is well known that those people at the top of the social hierarchy are healthier and live longer than those at the bottom of the social hierarchy.[13] In contrast, infant mortality rate is inversely associated with a state's economic health and its educational infrastructure.[14] Unemployment is linked to increased risks for heart disease, depression, and alcohol abuse. Because rates of death and disease follow racial lines, the life expectancy of black Americans is six and a half years shorter than that of white Americans. Compared to their white counterparts using a variety of measures, the health status of the black population has declined every year since 1984.[15]

Other studies show that people live longer in places where the income gap between the poorest and the richest is smallest. For example, Japan and Sweden rank first and second in the world in life expectancy and have the two lowest levels of income inequality. The Oglala Sioux and the U.S. homeless have a life expectancy of between fifty-five and fifty-nine years, worse than that of many third world countries.[16] Similarly, the death rate in Louisiana is 30 percent higher than it is in Utah, where the gap between rich and poor is less than Louisiana's.[17]

How societal determinants produce health is the subject of much debate. Traditionally, researchers posited that societal factors—gender, education, occupation, race, and so forth—work through a broad range of intermediate variables such as lifestyle, poverty, and genetic differences. The common interpretation was that the poor either are more prone to engage in risky behaviors—eating high-fat diets, smoking, being obese, having unsafe sex—or are deprived of some material condition, such as adequate health care or a safe environment.

The new evidence reasserts the sociologist Emil Durkheim's assumption that the community itself is an entity.[18] More complex than the sum of the individuals that make up its population, the community—the whole—acts on and through each person to influence the health status of each. The issue is not poverty per se but income inequality, for the evidence indicates that the magnitude of economic inequality between the people at the top and those at the bottom of the social ladder matters more than the absolute standard of living.

Durkheim was the first to posit that income inequality signifies a breakdown in the social fabric, which then leads to a loss of social stability and to individual feelings of anxiety, dissatisfaction, and disaffection. Researchers now know that over time these negative feelings can damage delicate neuroendocrine and immunological mechanisms, resulting in disease.

Recently, Ichiro Kawachi and Bruce Kennedy showed that *social capital*—trust, reciprocity, and mutual aid—are strongly correlated with overall mortality. To oversimplify a bit, people were asked whether they "bowled alone" or belonged to groups. When asked, "Can most people be trusted—or would most people try to take advantage of you if they got the chance?" both disaffection and distrust highly correlated with income inequality and with overall mortality.[19]

Similar findings attribute differences in health status to differences in autonomy, respect, and material resources.[20] Some of these links are easy to see. Material needs are the lowest level on Maslow's hierarchy, and trust is a component of safety—Maslow's second level of needs. The effect that respect and the power to pursue one's goals have on health status, however, is more difficult to see. Signifying esteem, the second-highest level in Maslow's hierarchy of needs, autonomy and respect are the hallmarks of inclusion. Bestowing a sense of worth, acknowledging that a person's contributions are valued, that he or she belongs, inclusion signifies the right to choose. Inclusion also denotes protection. For when we can claim as our own society's privileges and sanctions—potent social proscriptions against being taken advantage of for others' gains—we embody the very fabric of society.

In other words, those at the bottom end of the social ladder, given their druthers, would prefer to be free of economic worries; to live in a safe, clean, spacious environment with good schools and recreational facilities for their kids; and to have easy access to medical care and shopping. They'd like to be paid a living wage. Those at the bottom end of the wage scale take care of our kids, grow and package our food, and pave our streets. Even the outcome of a surgery depends, to some extent, on how carefully they clean the operating room.

Those at the low end of the wage scale, however, don't have the economic and political power to choose. They can't afford to live in communities where material resources are in abundance. They simply don't have the economic and political power to keep toxic waste sites out of their backyard, to prevent health insurers from redlining their occupations and geographic locations, or to live where it is safe for their kids to be outdoors.

Despite prevailing stereotypes of race and poverty, most people at the low end of the wage scale work hard and would make the right choices— if they could. The higher incidences of cancer, heart disease, violence, suicide, and substance abuse are found among the more vulnerable members of society because they *are* more vulnerable. The vulnerable are a good host for a multitude of intermediate variables because of their disadvantaged position. Given the disparity in income, those at the bottom of the social ladder have fewer choices and less autonomy. For autonomy, to a great extent, is bestowed by the norms, values, sanctions, privileges, and obligations that explain who is in and who is out.

In an era marked by cutthroat competition, trust and inclusion are in short supply. The irony is profound, for "the most important reason why more egalitarian societies are healthier seems to be they enjoy better social relationships."[21] There are more interpersonal trust, more helpfulness, and more friendship and less hostility, coercion, and violence. Also, there are fewer intrapersonal feelings of anxiety, inferiority, and inadequacy. In short, people are happier, and there is more social cohesion.

The challenge lies in the implementation of societal resources. Conceptually, societal resources are outside the biomedical model of health. Social structures—not discrete individuals—are the object of care, and interventions are social policies and programs. Aimed at advancing the health of the whole by ameliorating social and economic conditions, such policies tend to be at odds with traditional economic and political solutions.

Still, policies are the work of individuals and special interest groups, which means that the cultivation of trust and inclusion is an individual affair. Like love and belonging, respect and cooperation link people together reciprocally. In other words, trust and sharing the responsibility for the health of the whole is a two-way street. At one end, the cultivation of autonomy and respect commits the less well off to develop greater self-reliance. At the other end, we'd all be healthier if those who have more shared their power and resources with those who have less.

ENVIRONMENTAL DETERMINANTS OF HEALTH

Our environment is the geophysical space we inhabit. It is a kind of womb. Comprised of air, soil, water, and solar energy, the environment is the primary source of our basic physiological needs—food, shelter, clothing, air, and water. Thus it is a major determinant of health for individuals and communities. To the extent that people are deprived of any of the basic physiological needs, or that the environment is toxic or hazardous, health is adversely affected.

Environmental health hazards stem from a multitude of diverse causes. Scientists are just beginning to understand the link between human health and the quality of the environment. Noise; ozone depletion; global warming; habitat destruction; species extinction; and the poisoning of air, water, and soil by chemical toxins and radioactive waste are indicators of a deteriorating environment.

Ecosystem disruption is associated with outbreaks of Ebola virus. Lyme disease and Hanta virus have followed in the wake of suburban expansion. Chlorinated hydrocarbons, such as DDT and PCPs, are associated with cancer and birth defects. Lead, mercury, and other heavy metals are implicated in the etiology of heart disease, reproductive problems, cancer, and allergies. Upstream fertilizers, hormones, herbicides, pesticides, and heavy metals get into the food chain, resulting in a wide range of diseases.

Pollutants enter the body through food and water. We also breathe in pollutants through the air and absorb them through our skin. Once inside the body, these toxins can alter one or more of the body's organ systems. The immune, endocrine, reproductive, and central nervous systems seem to be particularly sensitive to assault, and children seem to be more sensitive than adults. A United Nations report cited in Erlich & Erlich shows that 14 million children die annually from causes related to environmental degradation.[22]

Although few still dispute the link between environmental quality and human health, the questions of when and how to intervene are keenly contested. Unlike the accident that results in a broken bone, the cause-and-effect relationship between environmental factors and health is not immediate. Toxic effects may occur years after initial exposure. Moreover, most environmental agents don't cause a specific disease or syndrome but a range of symptoms and diseases that seem to vary from individual to individual. Sickness that has a long induction period is further complicated because there may be more than one toxic agent at work. Variations in how much, how long, and which factors, technically known as the "total body load principle," make cause and effect difficult to determine. The relationship between environmental factors and health is neither simple nor linear.

Furthermore, the physiological effects of environmental pollutants can be exacerbated or buffered by social factors. For instance, Tokyo, which is one of the world's largest and most polluted cities, records the lowest infant mortality and longest life expectancy of any place on earth. In comparison, disease and mortality are generally high in socially disadvantaged populations living in polluted areas.[23]

Public health, occupational, and environmental medicine all claim responsibility for a healthy environment. The care of the environment as it is now structured does not actually belong to health care. For starters, the recipient of care is our geophysical habitat—the whole planet and the part where we live and work. This is a radical departure from biomedicine's conceptual framework of caring for individuals, one at a time.

Moreover, the resources used in the production of a healthy environment are policies and regulations. These resources are outside of health care's authority, for their jurisdiction primarily belongs to the Environmental Protection Agency (EPA) and the Occupational Safety and Health Administration (OSHA) or to international agreements, such as the Kyoto Accords. Thus the public's protection from environmental hazards is largely a function of law rather than health care.

Caring for the environment is fraught with challenges. For starters, not everyone sees the earth as our womb. Many do not perceive the earth as a living, breathing organism fed by solar energy, nor do they perceive the earth's crust, air, water, and its creatures as one self-regulating whole. Instead, many still perceive the earth as merely an inert deposit of natural resources to be consumed in the pursuit of economic growth and better standards of living. Many still perceive geopolitical boundaries as impermeable membranes, as though toxic waste dumped in your backyard won't eventually be carried by wind and rain into my backyard.

Thus policies and regulations aimed at protecting the environment and reducing environmental hazards are often at odds with traditional economic and political solutions. Our market economy, with its modes of production and consumerism lifestyle, contributes to pollution and environmental degradation. As a result, in order to protect ourselves from the metabolic damage caused by living in a toxic habitat, we would need to reduce what many of us consider a necessary standard of living. Finally, there's the challenge, What's in it for me? Compared to the immediacy of taking a pill, environmental influences are subtle, happen over a longer period of time, and often can be observed only at the population level.

Sometimes it is what we don't see that harms us the most, yet the relationship between health and the environment is real. Here, too, the relationship between healthy people and a healthy environment is continuous and reciprocal. Each one of us depends upon the environment for our most basic physiological needs. How we will care for our environment; whether we will continue to pollute it and profligately spend its raw materials or whether we will implement more stringent environmental policies and regulations is far from clear.

SPIRIT AND HEALTH

The spirit refers to nonmaterial forces of life. Like gravity, the spirit is intangible and is thought of as a kind of an omnipresent, subtle energy field that transcends the personal mind/body ensemble. Based on the assumption that we are spiritual beings in physical bodies, the purpose of care of the spirit is to help patients connect with something greater than themselves. Essentially, spiritual care refers to the use of touch, prayer, meditation, grace, scripture, music, spiritual imagery, and inner dialogue to support patients through their sickness, either back to recovery or through death.

The role of the spirit in health is controversial, because spirit is difficult to describe and even more difficult to research. For starters, the word *spirit* means different things to different people, and it goes against traditional body-as-machine beliefs. Moreover, spirit is impossible to grasp, measure, quantify, or see; it can't be isolated in a test tube or weighed on a scale. Being intangible, spirit can't be objectively studied or apprehended by contemporary technology. It's like wind. The best we can do is observe its effects.

Hundreds of scientific studies show that spirit is important to health. For instance, cardiac patients who were prayed for daily needed fewer medications, had fewer complications, and realized more desirable outcomes than those who were not prayed for.[24] Patients with strong religious faith were three times more likely to survive heart surgery than those without.[25] Meditation helps cancer patients find contentment and hope. The elderly who attended church regularly were found to be physically healthier and less depressed.[26] In short, epidemiological studies show that those who have faith in the transcendent tend to cope better, have fewer psychological problems, have better health in general, and survive longer than those who do not.

While the scientific studies are relatively new, the importance of spirit to health goes back to ancient times. Throughout history, the sick have used prayer, meditation, and scripture to allay suffering and have found symptom relief through the laying on of hands.

Reiki therapy and Therapeutic Touch (TT) are two modern versions of the laying on of hands. Both have philosophical roots steeped in Chinese and Ayurvedic medicine traditions. Nurses as well as therapists use TT and Reiki to relieve pain, decrease stress, allay emotional trauma, ease breathing, and accelerate wound healing. Knowledgeable practitioners are sensitive to differences of energy level and flow in the patient's energy field. Energy imbalances and sensations of congestion or depletion are noticed, and the intent of the practitioner is to rebalance the patient's energy field. Patients who received either of these therapies during surgery reported that they needed less anesthesia, had less postoperative pain, and recovered more quickly than other patients.[27]

Spirit, God, Qi, prana, and life force are the names typically given to this subtle energy. Practitioners believe that all humans embody this energy. Healing occurs because the energy can be focused and passed between people. The practitioner does not create the energy, only focuses it; nor does the practitioner control the outcome. The practitioner's conscious redirection of energy can only encourage the potential for the patient's own inherent capacity to heal.

While energy medicine is relatively new to Americans, the notion of spirit has long been central to allaying suffering. Suffering refers to mental and spiritual distress induced by a loss of integrity or cohesion. Identity and family relationships are frequently disrupted by chronic and life-threatening disease, and impending death usually disrupts all that is familiar. Such things as pain, fear, dependence on others, or even dietary changes can unravel familiar habits, self-identities, and civic responsibilities. Feeling the losses acutely, the patient suffers, as do the family and, usually, close friends.

Prayer, meditation, scripture, and hymns are known to reduce suffering for they connect us with a transcendental source signifying unity, meaning, and comfort. Offering hope, consolation, and guidance, prayer and scripture help repair torn relationships and remind us we are not alone. There is a kind of strength and wisdom in knowing that others, too, have been tested. Generally, when people feel supported by something greater than themselves, suffering abates. Spiritual care helps people to grieve their losses, deepen love, and reconcile broken relationships, though seldom to their preruptured state. Also, spiritual care helps patients and families find contentment and gratitude for what they have now—even though the sickness may be incurable or life threatening, and death may be imminent.

The role of the spirit in health is controversial and is clouded by polarized attitudes. At one extreme are the skeptics who criticize spiritual interventions as unscientific and bogus. At the other are the misguided who believe everything must be treated by prayer. In the middle, however, are enlightened practitioners—nurses, doctors, therapists, hospital chaplains, and hospice volunteers, to name just a few. Their goal is to heal. Healing takes place on many levels, not just in the body but in the mind and spirit and between the self and others. For these practitioners, health is not the absence of disease, nor is care synonymous with cure.

INPUTS AND OUTPUTS

So far in our inquiry, we have discovered two things. First, health is not static but is represented by a continuum of needs: prevention and acute, chronic, and life-threatening conditions. Second, health is generated by a continuum of determinants: societal, environmental, medical care, behav-

Table 4.1
Inputs, Outputs, and Objects of Care

Form of Care	Input	Output	Object of Care
Environmental	Air, water, food, shelter	Physical survival	Population
Societal	Respect and inclusion	Increased trust and helpfulness, safety	Population
Biomedicine	Drugs and surgery	Cure, control of symptoms	Individual physical bodies
Behavioral	Self-expression, self-regulation, self-care	Improved cognitive skills, adaptability, and coping skills	Individual minds
Relationships	Love and affection	Intimacy and inclusion	Patient and family
Spirit	Prayer, ritual, scripture, laying on of hands	Meaning, self-esteem; return to the transcendent	Individual spirit

ioral, biological, and genetic. These determinants represent the types of remedy or form of care that individuals and populations need to be healthy during a span that begins in utero and ends with death.

One question leads to another. Inquiry is a spiral process. It is not merely circling the same old issues. Instead, a spiral process indicates that the inquiry is penetrating deeper into the layers of thought. We could say that we are connecting our strategies and actions to our attitudes and beliefs, which we connect to even more abstract phenomena: cultural values and an organizing worldview. We have been accounting for the layers of thought that govern health care's effectiveness.

The results of our most recent inquiry raise another question: For health care to be more effective, which forms of care should belong to health care? This is a boundary-setting question, now approached from the insights laid out in Table 4.1.

HEALTHY SYSTEMS INTEGRATE

By definition, healthy systems integrate their parts. Because the parts cooperate to preserve the whole, healthy systems are stable systems. Health care, however, is not well integrated. It is an amalgam of conflicting policies and multiple delivery systems (public health, mental health, and biomedicine) that are further fragmented into multiple specialties and subspecialties. The social, environmental, behavioral, relational, and spiritual forms of care are either excluded from the clinical gaze or collapsed, reduced to medical technology. Equally significant, not everyone who's sick has access to care.

As long as we persist with a modern understanding, we will attempt to make the health care system more effective by tampering with our favorite broken part inside it. Using our best linear thinking, we will attempt to make care more effective by training more physicians and utilizing better technology: more potent drugs, genetic engineering, newer screening methods, and so forth. However useful, these improvements will not significantly increase health care's effectiveness. Training twice as many physicians doesn't make health care twice as effective; it merely raises the total cost of health care. Likewise, newer technology can neither relieve individual suffering nor redress the societal and environmental causes of disease that effect the health of whole populations.

However, if we change our mind and begin to embrace a postmodern view, a new understanding of health and care unfolds. We see health as capacity, referenced by a continuum of needs, and we see care as a continuum of remedies. As a result, we begin to see the interactions of the elements that generate the health care system. It is in the network of interactions that opportunities for better integration appear.

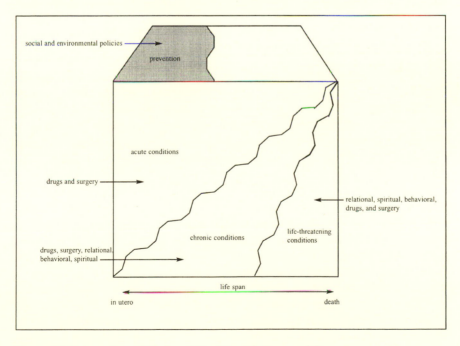

Figure 4.3 Integration of States of Health with Forms of Care

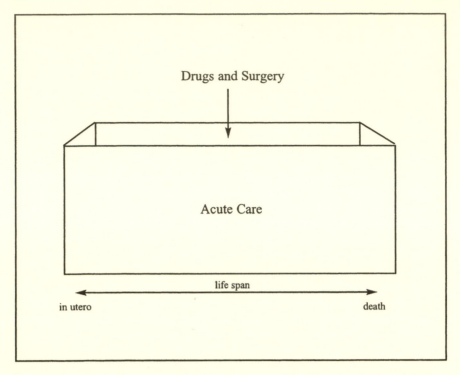

Figure 4.4 Needs and Remedies Collapsed into Acute Care and Medical Technology

In systems language, opportunities for better integration are known as high-leverage actions. High-leverage actions are system changes that lead to significant, enduring improvement, the essence of health care reform. As illustrated by Figure 4.3, high-leverage opportunities are at the boundaries between health needs. Leverage occurs by distinguishing each type of need in the continuum of life and then integrating this continuum with the appropriate forms of care. In comparison, the modern health care system, illustrated by Figure 4.4, largely collapses all needs into acute care and collapses all forms of care into medical technology, which is neither effective nor efficient.

Figure 4.3 represents the integration of the continuum of health needs with forms of care. By distinguishing the variety of health needs, health care's resources can be used more efficiently and effectively. Moreover, health care's resources can be distinguished from those that best belong to other social institutions. For example, drugs and surgery are the right care for a simple appendectomy, but the resource mix for childhood diabetes also includes behavioral and relationship resources. At the end of life, dignity, comfort, and support for patients and their families usually include more of the behavioral, relationship, and spiritual resources and less of biomedicine's technology. In contrast, prevention represents an economy of scale, and environmental and social resources are more important than medical technology.

The forms of care and the continuum of needs present a far more complex picture of health and care than the one presented by biomedicine. In this complex picture, biomedicine is only one of several determinants of health. This clearer and expanded understanding of health is in sharp contrast to the belief promoted by many of health care's dominant stakeholders that biomedicine is the primary determinant of health. Whether the entire continuum of resources—particularly the environmental and social determinants of health—rightfully belongs to health care is not clear and is beyond the scope of this book. The continuum, which certainly reveals the need for collaboration among the health care system and other social agencies, underscores the significance of the question, What is best for the nation's health?

INERTIA OF THE STATUS QUO

In systems language, improving a system's effectiveness requires changing a system's structure. Large-system change is difficult. Because large systems reflect, reproduce, and reinforce the status quo, it is their nature to resist change. So it's not surprising that despite more than thirty years of investigating the determinants of health, care of the sick remains mechanistic and fragmented. People aren't cared for as a whole.

The continued focus on the 20 percent of the determinants of health, the interventions sanctioned by health care, has as much to do with economic reasons as scientific reasons. On one hand, preference is given to research that unravels biological pathways that can be linked to the development of new technologies guaranteed to produce a quick return on investment. On the other hand, individuals are covered by health insurance, and the restrictions imposed by health plans present strong economic barriers to changing the system's structure.

FLOOD REDUX

Viewing health care through Flood's holistic prism, the question What is care? is an inquiry into health care's effectiveness. Effectiveness means doing the right thing. Part of our inquiry has involved asking ourselves whether biomedicine's notions of healer, patient, cause, and remedy result in an effective system. The smaller answer is yes, for health care is very effective at treating acute, episodic conditions. However, the larger answer is no: The health status of Americans ranks thirty-seventh in the world.

In this era of chronic diseases, health care still treats only one person at a time using high-tech cures. None of health care's interventions is directed toward redressing the causes that affect the health status of the whole population, and very few of health care's interventions are directed toward relieving suffering or the effective management of chronic disease.[28]

The second, and deeper, part of our inquiry concerned the elements the system should rightfully include in order to fulfill its purpose. On one hand, the inquiry exposed the influence health insurance—a powerful but generally silent element—has on quality and access to care, and it exposed the continuum of conditions for which people need care and the multiple forms of care, forms that are now available to some of the American public. On the other hand, the inquiry caused us to reexamine the purpose of health care. Inquiry is a recursive process, a spiraling through the depths of thought and a to-ing and fro-ing among the four questions until (1) the elemental answers are eventually congruent, and (2) we are satisfied that the health care system is coherent when we view it through Flood's prism. Regardless of where we are in this recursive process, ineluctably, the heart of the process is our answer to, What does it mean to care for fellow human beings?

QUESTIONS FOR THE READER

1. What kind of care do you expect from health care? What experiences and beliefs have helped form your views?

2. Referring to Maslow's hierarchy of needs, which of these resources are important to your health? What will these resources produce? Should these resources be paid for with tax dollars, by health insurance, or some other way?

3. What resources does your doctor use? To what extent does your health plan determine the kind of care you receive?

4. How do you care for yourself? Do you wait for something to happen and then seek medical attention, or do you have good health habits, a network of friends, live in a safe place, and have faith in something greater than yourself?

5. Do you rely on drugs and technology to make you feel better even if there is evidence that other interventions or changing your mind or your environment are more effective?

6. If you have a disability or a chronic disease, how is it cared for? What do you expect from your doctor? Do you put your faith in a medical cure? What responsibilities do other providers, such as social workers and psychologists, family, and friends, have regarding your care? What do you think they would say their responsibilities are?

7. Do you have the knowledge, financial resources, and support from your family and work to follow your doctor's orders? What resources might you need that are not covered by your health insurance?

8. If you have a life-threatening illness, do you expect the act of dying to be prolonged with whatever technology is available, regardless of cost or utility? Do you want to be kept comfortable and allow death to come naturally? Have you shared your expectations with your doctor and your family?

9. Where does health care end and other institutions/agencies—such as mental health services, churches, social services, OSHA, and so forth—begin?

10. What care do people with disabilities, chronic diseases, the frail elderly, and teenage mothers need?

11. How do you care for others if a compassionate response demands a redistribution of your time, wealth, power, or prestige?

12. Are you willing to care for people who are not like you or who don't like you? Are you willing to ensure that others have the benefits you choose for yourself?

CHAPTER 5

How Much Is Enough?

Medicine is a science of uncertainty, and an art of probability.
Sir William Osler

Just as What is care? was, in Flood's terms, an inquiry into health care's effectiveness, How much is enough? is an inquiry into health care's efficiency. In systems language, *enough* is shorthand for the amounts of resources, or inputs, the health care system uses to produce its output—health. Efficiency is asking whether the right amount of resources flow to the right recipients at the right time to achieve what is best for the nation's health. In short, efficiency refers to not wasting resources.

Questions of enough are questions of finitude; they implicitly assume there are limits to life as well as to resources. Enough indicates rationing, and rationing, which also refers to not wasting resources, implies limits to longevity, to health care's ability to cure, to technology's beneficence, and to the profits stakeholders can make. Questions of enough are complex, confusing, and emotionally charged because our answers to How much is enough? will (1) affect each system in the nested hierarchy of systems, and (2) affect all of health care's stakeholders, albeit differently.

Inquiry is like rock climbing in that the next move depends upon the present position. Moving through thought, so to speak, our answers to How much is enough? largely depend upon what we have learned from our inquiry into What is health? and What is care? Because our inquiry is actually a search for coherence, it follows that our answers to How much is enough? should balance with our answers to What is health? and What is care? We are searching for information that will, in Flood's terms, generate an effective, efficient, and fair health care system.

WE HAVE THE MOST

In Chapter 1, we saw that health care economics is best described as a continuous, circular quest to maximize utility. The patients' goal is to maximize health, while the goal of the other stakeholders is to maximize profits. We also saw that by pulling new goods and services into health care, third-party reimbursement and federal funding mechanisms reinforce health care's economic expansion.

Pulled by third-party reimbursement and federal funding, per capita spending on technology increased 791 percent in the United States between 1960 and 1995. Likewise, hospital beds proliferated due to easy access to large amounts of capital from Medicare agreements and the Hospital Survey and Construction Act of 1946, also known as the Hill-Burton Act, a federal program providing hospital construction funds. Although the number of hospital beds began dropping in the 1980s, with occupancy rates below 63%[1], the United States has more hospital beds than it needs.

Since 1960, the number of physicians has nearly tripled, from 251,200 to 704,700. The number of physicians per population went from around 735 persons per physician to about 369 persons per physician between 1960 and 2000.[2] During this period, physician income rose sharply, from an average of $12,000 in 1950 to $42,000 in 1970 to $190,000 in 1997. In comparison, the average annual wage for Americans was $27,426 in 1997.[3]

Other types of provider also proliferated during this period. The number of registered nurses more than doubled, from 592,000 in 1960 to 1,272,900 in 1980, and it doubled again by 2000.[4] Ironically, despite the growth in numbers, the nursing population is aging. The present average age of nurses is forty-five, and fewer than 10 percent are younger than thirty. New occupations also emerged, including physician assistant, respiratory therapist, quality assurance auditor, and others. By 1993, health care was second only to the retail trade in number of workers, accounting for 7.3 percent of the total workforce.

Finally, the number of insurance companies also increased during this forty-year period, reaching about 1,400 companies in the mid-1990s. Within the realm of insurance, managed care—the purported answer to soaring costs—not only did not contain costs but significantly increased health care's bureaucratic burden. It is estimated that bureaucracy accounts for roughly 30 percent of total health care costs.[5] To illustrate, our largest HMOs keep 20–25 percent of premiums for their overhead and profit.[6] In comparison, the overhead for Canada's National Health Insurance (NHI) is 1 percent,[7] and Medicare's is roughly 4 percent.[8] Woodhandler and Himmelstein have estimated that were the huge amounts of red tape and paperwork and other administrative costs reduced to Canadian levels, at least $120 billion would be saved annually, enough to adequately insure both underinsured and uninsured Americans.[9]

The United States has the most expensive health care system in the world. We have more doctors, more hospital beds, more technology, and more insurance companies than most other countries. Despite having more of everything, including more uninsured citizens, more Americans are dissatisfied with their health care system than are European and Canadians.

MOST ISN'T BEST

According to Paul Starr, the spending gap between the United States and other countries is not due primarily to our high volume of high-tech care (see Table 5.1). Rather, when compared to Canada—the second-highest spender and the country whose system is most similar to the United States'—between a third and a half of the gap is due to higher administrative and insurance costs in the United States. Roughly another third reflects the greater number of diagnostic tests U.S. physicians order and the higher fees U.S. physicians charge.[10]

Compared with other countries, the United States provides far more cardiac surgery and organ transplants. However, it provides less primary and preventive care. The British do fewer tests and less renal dialysis and cardiac surgery, have fewer intensive care beds, and are less likely to treat cancer that is not highly responsive to chemotherapy. While hip replacement surgery and chemotherapy for potentially curable tumors are essentially the same in both countries, Great Britain spends more on children—119 percent per adult spending compared with the United States' 37 percent.[11]

Table 5.1
How the United States Stacks Up Internationally

	health care spending per capita	inpatient days per capita	physician contacts per capita	infant mortality per 1,000 live births	life expectancy at birth M	life expectancy at age 80 (M)	% populatio n age 65 and older	% public dissatisfied ±
U.S.	$2,354	1.3	5.3	10.	71.5	6.9	12.3	90
Canada	$1,683	2.0	6.6	7.2	73.	6.9	11.1	40
Germany	$1,232	3.5	11.5	7.6	71.8	6.1	15.4	45
Japan	$1,035	4.1	12.9	4.8	75.5	6.9	11.2	?
Britain	$836	2.0	4.5	9.0	72.4	6.4	15.6	65
OECD average for 24 nations	$1059	2.8	6.0	10.6	72.1	6.3	13	

± Data from Harvard-Harris-ITF Ten-Nation Survey, 1990; Organization for Economic Cooperation and Development.
Source: Starr, P. (1994). *The Logic of Health-Care Reform.* New York: Whittle Books, p. 18.

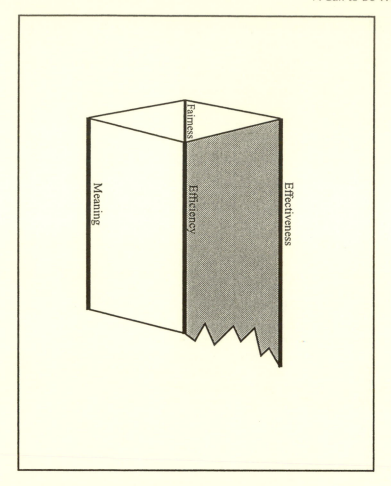

Figure 5.1 Efficiency and Effectiveness Are Out of Alignment

Although Britain spends less per capita than other industrial countries, 65 percent of British are dissatisfied with their health care system. In contrast, Americans spend the most but 90 percent of Americans are dissatisfied with health care. Despite the common wisdom You get what you pay for, Americans aren't as healthy as the Japanese, Canadians, or Europeans. Americans rank twenty-fourth worldwide in life expectancy and twenty-second in infant mortality. When compared to other industrialized countries, the United States has more cancer, more coronary disease, more violence, and a more severe HIV epidemic.[12]

Using Flood's terms, we'd say efficiency and effectiveness are way out of alignment. Schematically, our very expensive system looks like Figure 5.1.

HOW WE GOT TO WHERE WE ARE

When it comes to health care, we truly are like the fabled blind men and the elephant. Americans don't all see the same health care system. Different stakeholders have different images of health care, have different turf to protect, and are inconsistent in their use of modern versus postmodern concepts. Essentially, the public has a modern view of health, of health as a state of perfection, and a postmodern view of care.

From a systems perspective, our understandings of health and care contribute to health care's inefficiency. As uneven legs on a stool preclude stability, our understanding of health and of care precludes coherent answers to enough. The former implies unlimited health and the latter, an unlimited market basket of health care goods and services. Together, they reinforce the illusion of no limits: that sickness, aging, and death can be defeated by medical technology; that next quarter's profits will always be greater.

If we inquire more deeply, however, we see a potent, silent force driving the prevailing understanding of health, care, and enough. Buried deep within our psyche is what Ernest Becker refers to as an existential fear of death and decay. "This deep fear leaves us hopelessly absorbed with ourselves. If we care about anyone it is usually ourselves first of all."[13] Becker claims that our fear of death has to do with a struggle for self-esteem. His basic arguments are that we have been conditioned to feel that our own life is not enough because our unique and personal contributions are seldom valued, and that we are afraid of revealing who we really are. As a result, we become selfish and seek to bolster our self-esteem by amassing material goods. We compensate by denying death and amassing wealth.

Basically, Becker is saying that we are trapped in our fear that there's not enough because we don't know how to be *real* to one another—to appreciate one another as biological, psychological, social, and spiritual beings; however, for existence to be truly human is to make peace with life's limitations. The remainder of this chapter explores the actions we've taken to either make peace or avoid making peace with life's limitations.

OUR FEAR OF DEATH

In 1984, Richard Lamm, then governor of Colorado, made the headlines, allegedly saying that the elderly have a duty to die and get out of the way. Although brusque, Lamm voiced three implicit but prevailing assumptions: There are not enough health care dollars to provide care for both the old and the young. There are not enough health care dollars to provide high-tech care for the elderly and basic services for the poor and young. Finally, death comes only to the elderly. Essentially, these three assumptions are a tacit argument that age is the obvious criteria for health care rationing.

Certainly, much of the economic focus has been on the elderly. The United States spends about 10 percent of its health care dollars on the elderly in their last year of life. Nearly 30 percent of Medicare dollars are spent on the 5 percent of its enrollees who die in a given year, and 40 percent of these expenditures occur in the last month of life.[14]

Age by itself, however, is a poor prognostic indicator, and not only the elderly have expensive end-of-life care. Other research shows that for all ages, 18 percent of health care dollars are spent for care given in the last year of life, three-quarters of it in the last month. Health care's expenses are only part of the picture, for end-of-life care is also very costly to families. Thirty-one percent of families deplete their life savings, 40 percent are pushed into poverty, and 20 percent of those who care for sick family members while trying to work end up losing their jobs.[15]

Although costs are serious concerns, the focus on economics eclipses the deeper moral questions, such as who decides when the end is near, and who decides what are the right kind and amount of care. Once, people were more resigned to death, but with the scientific ability to develop ever-more-sophisticated drugs, implant prosthesis, transplant organs, and splice genes comes the fantasy of immortality—a cure for cancer, an end to birth defects, morbidity compressed into the very end of a very long life. Such societal expectations continue to eclipse any notion of enough. Afraid of death, "we deny the only outcome our lives can possibly have."[16]

Consequently, technology has become a Faustian bargain. Blood transfusions and antibiotics can buy a little more time for disease-ravaged bodies. Tube-feedings, kidney dialysis, and mechanical ventilation can maintain patients long after the body has lost the ability to eat, eliminate waste, or breathe for itself. Having reduced life to discrete, measurable events that can be treated by technology, however briefly or uselessly, the prevailing rule of thumb is: If available, life-sparing technology should be used, as long as the patient has insurance.

Partially—because death cannot be predicted with 100 percent certainty—patients and physicians find themselves entangled in technology's moral dilemma. Withdrawing treatment seems like killing; continued support prolongs dying. Meanwhile, fears of morphine-induced respiratory failure and misplaced fears of addiction cause many patients to spend their final days in agonizing pain. With technology the only solution, no wonder physician-assisted suicide is seriously considered.

PLANNING AHEAD, THE PATIENT NEEDS TO LEAD

By denying their eventual mortality, patients tacitly surrender their autonomy to their physician. During the dominance of fee-for-service reimbursement, physicians tended to use any treatment needed for survival. So strong was this cultural value that the Karen Quinlan and Nancy

Cruzan families had to sue for the right to terminate their daughters' care. Since these trials, the patients' right to choose has been a value sanctioned by the courts, but the values are once again changing, albeit silently, as managed care has made physicians more cost-conscious. Unless a patient has clearly expressed, in advance, a wish for life-saving treatment, physicians tend toward providing less-intensive care to patients with sicknesses that appear to be fatal—especially if the patient is elderly or poor or doesn't have family members at the bedside.

The problem is largely *not* the withdrawal of intensive care but that other forms of care that provide comfort and support at the end of life— such as hospice and palliative care—are not offered. Despite the 1990 OBRA law that requires all health care agencies to inform adult patients about their right to accept or refuse treatment, most patients never fill out advance directive forms. Surrendering his autonomy, the patient waits for the doctor to initiate the conversation. Struggling with his or her own fears of death—for physicians have been trained to see death as their failure and an indicator of their clinical competency—the physician waits for the patient to initiate the conversation.

For a host of reasons, very few patients plan ahead. Planning ahead certainly has nothing to do with suicide or even implies that much about the end of life can be forecast with any certainty. Instead, planning ahead means to wonder, to meditate on life's impermanence. Planning ahead is to confront our fears forthrightly, to wonder what kinds of sickness should be intensively treated and what kinds should not and to contemplate the kinds of support and comfort measures that might be needed—or wanted—to relieve distressing symptoms when intensive treatment is not the goal. It also means sharing one's concerns and wishes with one's family and physician. By asserting his or her own autonomy, the patient frees him- or herself and, paradoxically, frees the physician from the thrall of science and technology.

CAUGHT ON THE HORNS OF A DILEMMA

Our fear of death, our hopes for technology, and our faith in the ability of science to unravel the mysteries of the physical body tap into two very deep fears. Seemingly polar opposites, one is the fear of not enough health care, that care will be too little, too late, denied, inadequate, ineffective, or unaffordable. The other is the fear of too much, that death will be prolonged, painful, impersonal, and leave the family bankrupt.

As we've seen repeatedly, more technology is not necessarily better. The overuse of technology can cause as many or more adverse affects as its misuse or underuse. Moreover, society's great optimism about technology comes at the expense of so-called soft solutions, relational, societal, behavioral, and environmental.

Related to these fears of too little and too much is another dilemma, the fear of health care rationing. The primary fears are that premium costs will rise and/or health needs won't be met. Yet these fears are coming to pass for more and more Americans.

The word *dilemma* originally referred to a rhetorical device in which an opponent was presented with two alternatives. It didn't matter which one he chose, he lost the argument either way. One horn of the bull, so to speak, was as damaging as the other horn. We know we're caught when we tell ourselves that if we continue to operate this way, the situation will *get* worse, but that if we intervene, we'll *make* it worse —we are damned if we do and damned if we don't.

Because it is the nature of a dilemma to present only two alternatives, each of which is damaging or difficult, dilemmas keep things stuck. There seems to be no way out. Actually, there is no resolution at the level of thinking where the choices are offered. One of the gifts of inquiry is that in thinking about our thinking, we can discern layers of thought. There is a hierarchy of thought: data, assumptions, values, meaning, and an overarching worldview. Each level represents a higher level of abstraction. Like steps on a ladder, each level includes its predecessor and presents its unique set of qualities for interpreting our world. The higher we go, the more fully we understand our experiences—and the more choices we have. This is a long way of saying that dilemmas can be solved at a higher level of abstraction, but they cannot be solved at the level where they occur.

As long as rationing is presented as an economic issue, we are stuck in a game of economic musical chairs. The way out is to leave modernity's horns. Unlike Buddhism and other Eastern traditions, which treat morals and measures as two aspects of one phenomenon, the Western world, in accordance with Cartesian thought, treats morals and measures as two separate phenomena. Accordingly, health care tends to things that can be measured. Science is perceived as objective, or value-free. Having declared quantifiable data more real than subjective qualities, we let numbers trump morals.

Although rationing is presented as an economic issue, at a higher level of abstraction it is also a moral issue. At this level, rationing is a commitment to both economic efficiency and a predetermined level of care for each citizen. It's the balance point between too little and too much. In the best of all possible worlds, rationing strategies do not simply limit access to acute care but allocate resources across a spectrum of health needs: prevention and acute, chronic, and life-threatening conditions.

VICIOUS CYCLES

Dilemmas are to thought as vicious cycles are to systems. This isn't surprising, for thought is manifest in form. A vicious cycle is like an ava-

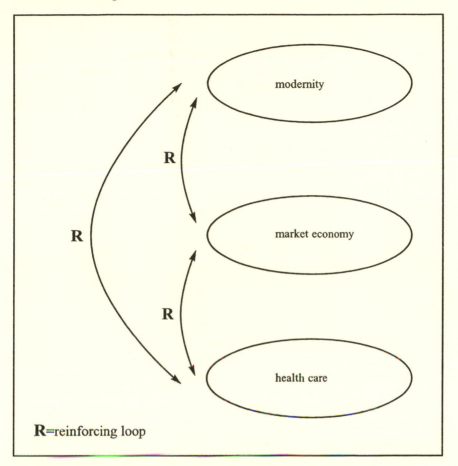

Figure 5.2 Feedback Loops among Modernity, the Market Economy, and Health Care Generate Multiple, Interlocking Vicious Cycles

lanche; it is a set of conditions that repeatedly multiply themselves. As the name *vicious cycle* implies, there is no way out, because the output of one stage becomes the input of the next. Each round builds, or amplifies, its predecessor, just as an avalanche grows in speed and size as it slides down a mountain. Seen as a schematic (Figure 5.2), there are too many reinforcing loops and too few balancing loops.

The irony is painful. Although health care emerges from and is informed by the modern worldview, which causes us to see systems as independent, the fact that we know this means that we are looking at health care and modernity through postmodern eyes. Yet we continue to hang on to modernity, which keeps us trapped in a vicious cycle of escalating costs. By assuming that science can control nature, we reinforce the illusion of no limits: that life will go on forever; that next quarter's profits will always be greater.

The reinforcing feedback loop between modernity and health care forms an airtight seal between the two systems, an impenetrable barrier to outside influences. Modernity reinforces the notion that sickness is simply a broken body part, which health care neatly reinforces with promises of ever-better technology and its claims of scientific cures.

Likewise, modernity traps us in a vicious cycle of unbridled economic growth. Reinforcing free market ideology and values, the feedback loop promotes unlimited economic growth. Adding insult to injury, the reinforcing feedback loop between the market economy and health care accelerates the rise in health care costs. Success is measured by surpassing last quarter's profits, and, like all other businesses, health care expects its profits to grow. Growth is achieved by raising prices, entering new markets, and reducing production costs. As demonstrated in chapter 1, the most efficient way to make money is to reduce production costs; consequently, efficiency has been pursued by tampering with processes inside of health care: deselecting the sick and the poor, denying and delaying care, and eliminating services that are costly to provide—behaviors contradictory to taking care of people.

Conditioned by modernity to see systems as separate, we don't see that health care spending is totally without brakes. We are blind to the fact that an economic balancing loop is missing. Without the addition of a balancing loop between our health care and our economic systems, strategies purported to make the health care system more effective are destined not just to fail but to exacerbate health care's soaring costs and diminishing returns.

For other businesses, the balancing loop is the free market's self-correcting mechanisms. These mechanisms don't and can't work for health care. On the supply side, entry isn't free. One can't simply become a provider or an HMO. On the demand side, employers and the government, not patients, typically purchase health plans; patients don't have complete information about price and quality but depend upon doctors to shop for them. On the supply side, again, physicians, not patients, determine the type and volume of care the patient receives. Moreover, a free market disciplines all players equally, but in health care, those most in need of services are the most vulnerable to exclusion, for they are the most costly.

It's not an accident that health care costs rose with Medicare and rose again with managed care. In the absence of a balancing loop between the market economy and health care, health care costs can only increase. The vouchers and medical savings accounts—solutions the George W. Bush administration is now proposing—can't contain costs, but will result in more of the same. Assuming the parts are independent, we continue to reinforce the illusion that each group of stakeholders is free to maximize its own self-interest.

Because the modern worldview conditions us to see separate parts rather than wholes, we don't connect the dots. We spend about 14 percent of our GDP on a system that contributes about 20 percent to the health status of the population because we don't see that health care and our market economy are connected *only* by a reinforcing loop.

We can't begin to address cost and quality issues as long as we continue to embrace modern assumptions. We can't afford to presume that health care is an independent system, disconnected from our economic system. Such blindness perpetuates the vicious cycle in which economic growth is reinforced, not checked. We can't afford to assume the stakeholders are independent or that money and morals are independent phenomena. Nor can we assume that health is the absence of disease and quality is perfection: a state of complete physical, mental, and social well-being (the WHO definition of health). Perfection is not for mortals; life and economic resources have their limits.

HEALTH CARE RATIONING

To control health care costs, all countries employ some form of rationing. For Americans, rationing usually has an ominous connotation. It conjures up negative images of government intervention, inferior quality, loss of personal choice, and exclusion. In systems language, however, rationing has to do with assuring that the right resources in the right amounts go to the right recipient at the right time. That's efficiency.

In actuality, all nations ration health care, although the methods vary. Rationing is achieved either through pricing and ability to pay or by limiting services. Moreover, rationing occurs either implicitly or explicitly. Most developed countries explicitly ration health care by limiting health care services. The United States, however, implicitly rations health care. (The one exception is the state of Oregon, which has an explicit rationing plan for its Medicaid population.)[17]

GLOBAL BUDGETS

As a commitment to both economic efficiency and a predetermined level of health care for each citizen, global budgets are an explicit form of rationing used by most developed countries. Simply speaking, a global budget is a balancing loop between the health care system and the economic system. Global budgets balance values.

Briefly, a global budget is a predetermined pool of monies tied to some arbitrary criterion, such as a fixed percentage of GDP or a fixed annual growth rate. Similar to a household budget but on a larger scale, the monies are allotted to such things as salaries, construction, and the purchase of medical technology. Because services are universally limited, medical care depends upon a professional assessment of medical need rather than the individual's ability to pay.

The financing of this pool of monies and how it is regulated varies from country to country. Generally, global budgets are financed through some sort of tax, and there are several levels of regulation. At the policy level, the government or a statutory entity establishes price controls, expenditure caps, and the types and location of services. At the local level, access to care depends upon the number and types of physicians and facilities. The doctor determines the patients' medical needs at the clinical level. The bottom line, however, guarantees the entire population access to a predetermined level of care. Equity of care, access, and cost control are the principle values of this form of rationing.

In countries that use global budgets, cuts in one area are justified on the grounds that money will be spent on other, higher-priority services. For example, Great Britain chooses to spend less money on high-tech, intensive care and relatively more money on childhood immunizations and palliative care for the terminally ill. So that universal access is affordable, Britain chooses not to fund excess capacity, even though waiting lists for nonurgent diagnostic tests and elective surgeries are the trade-offs.

Briefly, services are rationed through expenditure caps that control the types, geographic location, and volume of services. For example, the reason that Britain uses less surgery and has fewer ICU days, fewer hospital days in general, and fewer diagnostic tests is that these services are not readily available. Seeking a healthy balance between high-tech, acute care and the less costly palliative and preventive forms of care, the British have neither the excess high-tech capacity to drive its utilization nor the financial incentives to provide superfluous services. This is because the salaries of British physicians are also controlled; whereas the incomes of their American counterparts are directly related to utilization of resources.

To control *total* costs, prices are also controlled. Price controls maintain health care's affordability for lower-income families and prevent profiteering in a market where supply has been brought below demand. Essentially, price ceilings and expenditure caps work together, comprising a kind of check and balance. Expenditure caps ration care to patients, while price ceilings ration the profits that can be made by providers and the purveyors of health care's goods and services.

British drug costs are a good example of this check-and-balance function. In Britain, drugs cost two to ten times less than the same drugs cost in the United States. Not only do price ceilings control the sale price, but by law British drug companies can't spend more than 12 percent of their revenue on marketing and advertising. In comparison, Americans spend as much as 35 cents for every dollar of cost to pay for a drug's advertising. Likewise, U.S. drug expenditures have risen about 17–20 percent annually since 1970, from $5.5 billion in 1970 to $37.7 billion in 1990 to $61.1 billion in 1995 to an estimated $110–120 billion in 2000.[18]

The sharp rise in pharmaceutical prices coincided with the U.S. shift to managed care. Drug benefits are a reinforcing loop. More Americans with drug benefits means more access to drugs—because the insurer is picking up most of the tab. Just as reimbursement incentives for technology subsidize both supply and demand, pharmaceutical benefits reinforced the steep pharmaceutical price hikes of the 1990s. Before managed care, drugs were priced at what people typically could pay out of their own pockets, a kind of informal balancing loop. But managed care reinforced the pull of newer and ever-more-expensive drugs into the market, for the payer picked up most of the tab. This was good for patients with drug benefits because their co-pay capped their out-of-pocket costs; but it was very costly overall.

As the pharmaceutical example shows, unchecked growth has its own unrequited costs. In a system bereft of economic balancing loops, sooner or later all stakeholders pay the price. Patients without pharmaceutical benefits either pay the soaring retail prices or don't have their prescriptions filled, and in keeping with managed care's rising drug costs, everyone now pays higher insurance premiums. High costs, indeed, for the lack of systemic balancing loops.

In systems language, the significance of a global budget is that it is a series of complex economic balancing loops among the elements inside health care and between health care and the market economy. In short, a global budget provides the currently missing balancing loop between health care and the market economy. In addition, inside the health care system, a global budget assures an efficient distribution of resources among health care's parts.

Ideally, this multilayered set of interlocking mechanisms checks and balances cost, quality, and access. Of course, this presupposes (1) a belief that all citizens should have access to a predetermined level of care, and (2) congruent, coherent answers to What is health? and What is care? Simply put, global budgets check and balance the needs of one stakeholder group with the needs of the whole by rationing profits, salaries, and services. Price ceilings and expenditure caps balance profits and patient care, and other regulations are in place to assure quality. Because the health care budget is a fixed pool of monies, total costs are controlled and access is universal—like our access to roads, police, and fire protection. Tying the budget to a fixed percentage of the GDP or other annual growth rate prevents other aspects of our civic infrastructure—such as public safety, environmental protection, and education—from being eclipsed by runaway health care costs.

AMERICANS FEAR RATIONING

Historically, the powerful stakeholders have exploited the public's fears to maintain their own competitive edge. In the late 1990s, Citizens for Better Medicare, a front for the drug industry, derailed the proposed Medicare pharmaceutical plan with a television commercial in which good ole "Flo" said "keep the government out of my medicine cabinet." Similarly, the infamous "They choose. We Loose." ads sponsored by Health Insurance Association of America (HIAA) were instrumental in turning the public against the Clinton plan.

Medicare, which was vehemently opposed by the AMA, rations access on the basis of age. It is a program senior citizens feel entitled to and need. Today, nearly 40 million Americans depend on Medicare for their health care. Due to escalating costs and the increasing number of elderly, Medicare is forecast by some to be bankrupt in the year 2008. Some kind of reform is needed, or Medicare won't be available for the huge number of baby boomers who become eligible for it in 2011.

It's not at all clear how Medicare will be reformed—Medicare reform is not synonymous with health care reform and Medicare is only one part of the U.S. health care system—or how Medicare will ration care to elderly Americans. What *is* clear is that other industrialized countries spend less money on health care and have longer life expectancy—and larger elderly populations. For example, in the United States, in 1991 the population sixty-five years old and older was 12.6 percent of the total population, but it was 12.8 percent in Japan, 15 percent in Germany and France, 15.4 percent in the United Kingdom, and 17.9 percent in Sweden (see Table 5.2).

Without some form of global budget, decreased spending on the elderly can't be traded for access to care, or even traded for lower costs in general. Nor can decreased spending on intensive, end-of-life-prolonging medical care for the elderly be traded for hospice and palliative care at the end of life, because the trade-offs can only occur in the presence of a fixed budget and some notion regarding a reasonable length of life—a life span beyond which it is unreasonable to expect others to make expensive contributions. Without a fixed budget, it is impossible to determine where any cost savings would go. Without clear ideas regarding a reasonable length of life, there are no boundaries. Claims for resources are vague and open-ended; all death seems premature.

Other industrialized countries' lower health care costs and their better longevity and infant mortality rates validate explicit rationing. Still, rationing is very difficult for both U.S. health care professionals and the American public to address because explicit rationing contradicts the prevailing belief that health care is readily available to those in need. Also, explicit rationing understandably plays into people's fears of exclusion and loss.

Table 5.2
Health Expenditures, Life Expectancy, and Percentage of Elderly, Selected Countries

	Share of GDP (1991)	Life Expectancy (1993)	% Elderly (1991)
United States	13.4	75.8	12.6
France	9.1	78.0	15.0
Germany	8.5	76.1	15.0
Japan	6.8	79.2	12.8
Sweden	8.6	78.1	17.9
United Kingdom	6.6	76.5	15.4

Source: Stewart, C. T. (1995). *Healthy, Wealthy, or Wise: Issues in American Health Care Policy.* Armonk, NY: M.E. Sharpe, pp. 10–11.

DE FACTO RATIONING

We Americans largely believe that our health care system is free of rationing. This is an erroneous belief, however, because Americans experience extensive de facto health care rationing. Health care *is* rationed, even though we don't like to acknowledge it. Insurance coverage, geographic location, income, ethnicity, age, and the presence of preexisting medical conditions are all forms of de facto rationing.

In contrast to explicit rationing, which affects all citizens similarly, de facto rationing affects access and quality quite differently for different Americans. Due to our fears of explicit rationing and our habit of de facto rationing, Americans are sadly lacking any kind of consensus regarding (1) how much is enough, and (2) who has the authority to decide how care should be rationed. Consequently, de facto rationing is in the hands of special interest groups.

Unlike their European and Canadian counterparts, Americans do not have universal access to health care. According to one estimate, a million patients are denied care for economic reason annually.[19] Basically, this means that they do not have health insurance, or they have Medicare or Medicaid but cannot find a provider that accepts this insur-

ance, or they live in an inner city or rural region where health care services are in short supply. More than 20 million Americans are without
access to care because their region is either too poor or too sparsely pop-
ulated to support sufficient numbers of providers or adequate health
care facilities.

Moreover, in the United States, the amount and quality of care varies by
gender, ethnicity, and ability to pay. For instance, fewer women than men
have coronary-artery bypass surgery. African Americans do not receive the
same intensity of health care services as whites. The racial difference persists even when there are no incentives to treat one group ahead of another.
For example, both groups are covered by managed care,[20] Medicare,[21] or
treated in Veterans Administration hospitals.[22]

In comparison, the very wealthy have access to an unlimited array of
goods and services. Even when resources are scarce, those with enough
fame and fortune can bypass medical guidelines and skip to the front of
the line, which is what the ballplayer Mickey Mantle did when he received
a new liver. For those at the other end of the wealth-and-celebrity spectrum, the intensity and the quality of care are poorer. For instance, the in-
hospital death rate for the uninsured is 1.2 to 3.2 times higher than it is for
those with insurance; research attributes this to inadequate or delayed
access to care and inferior quality of care.[23]

Health insurance, too, is another form of de facto rationing. In fact,
health insurance is the United States' primary form of de facto rationing.
Access to care is difficult for people who don't have health insurance or
who can't afford its co-payments and deductibles. However, insurers also
ration goods and services by so-called bedside rationing and, because the
United States does not have a minimum standard of covered benefits, by
the wide variation in types and amounts of covered benefits among the
multitude of health plans.

BEDSIDE RATIONING

The shift from fee-for-service to managed care financing has led to what
is known as *bedside rationing*. An implicit form of rationing, bedside
rationing is distinguished from other forms in that rationing occurs
through the physician's clinical decisions. Through utilization review
practices and economic contracting, managed care has tied physicians'
income to their clinical decisions. Thus, if the care they deliver is judged
too expensive, physicians are financially penalized. In other words, bedside rationing is more than having the health plan dictate the type and
amount of goods and services it will pay for. It means that physicians' clinical decisions are influenced by the health plan.

Bedside rationing takes place along a continuum of varied economic
and moral values. At one end, bedside rationing is done in direct response
to financial incentives or disincentives. For example, a doctor may pre-

scribe a generic drug even if the brand name is more effective, or may use a less-durable hip prosthesis in a patient who is older than eighty but still very active. At the other end, rationing is the careful eschewing of high-tech, death-prolonging therapy. Examples include not placing an Alzheimer's patient with pneumonia on a ventilator or forgoing CPR on a young adult ravaged by HIV.

In the middle of this continuum lies a Gordian knot, a complicated conundrum of moral and economic values and clinical issues. The least-complicated decisions include those regarding forgoing the routine use of generic drugs and expensive tests when the probability of significant diagnostic information is low. For instance, there's widespread agreement that not ordering an MRI for a headache when the physiological exam is normal is the right use of resources, as are prescribing beta-blockers for all heart attack survivors and providing routine screening for colon cancer for people aged fifty and older. The care is cost-effective; that is, the tests and treatments result in a good outcome at a low cost.

The more complicated issues involve referrals and the use of treatment that is much more expensive and perhaps less effective. For example, a primary care physician may set a simple wrist fracture rather than refer the patient to an orthopedic surgeon. When the outcome significantly affects the patient, the decision becomes morally complex. Should the primary care doctor set the wrist to avoid financial penalties? What if the wrist belongs to a concert violinist? At what functional level should care be pegged? Is what is good for the meat cutter, good for the violinist? Who should decide?

Few ethical questions are raised when care that is of dubious value or unnecessary is withheld. However, when potentially beneficial services are withheld, serious ethical questions result. What is right when the mother of three young children who is life-threateningly ill with breast cancer wants a bone marrow transplant? Should her insurance company pay for her to receive the transplant, when some data suggest that the transplant is her best remaining hope, but other data indicate that the treatment's effectiveness is unproven?

On the other side of this argument, how would we feel about an insurance company spending its money on someone we disliked or whose behavior we disapproved? Would we want our premiums spent on a liver transplant for a known alcoholic, for instance? Who should decide how much is enough? Should it be the doctor, the insurance company paying for the care, courts of law, the patient, politicians, or society? How can any stakeholder group's decisions be fair, especially when there is a lack of consensus regarding health and care?

MANAGED CARE AND DE FACTO RATIONING

Managed care is now lobbying for legislative changes that will give it even more authority in determining what is medically necessary. If these changes are enacted, the ill-defined term *medically necessary* would give managed care more authority to ration covered benefits and to step up bedside rationing. It would also make it more difficult for patients to sue their health plans.

Justification for more authority to more tightly manage utilization is based on two interrelated notions. First, health insurance is unlike other insurance because health insurance is subject to moral hazard, and suppliers induce the demand. Second, not all care that is now provided is beneficial.

Moral hazard is the tendency to utilize more health care because a third party pays for it—a hazard to which both doctors and patients are subject. For instance, studies show that patients with comprehensive health insurance use almost one-third more health services than those with large deductibles.[24] The patient is only partially culpable, since suppliers also induce demand. For instance, it's widely believed that at least 20–30 percent of all medical procedures physicians do are probably unnecessary and, therefore, wasteful. Similarly, 8–86 percent of the surgeries performed annually have been found to be unnecessary and have caused substantial avoidable death and disability.[25]

Managed care is not morally neutral, however. Managed care is subject to the other side of the moral hazard coin. It puts physicians under great economic pressure to contain medical costs, for there is an inverse relationship between managed care's profits and the patients' utilization of services. The fewer medical services its covered population consumes, the more managed care's profits increase.

Of equal moral importance is access to care. About 43 million Americans don't have health insurance, and another 38 million are inadequately insured. This means that about a third of the public do not even seek out health care because they can't afford it. The brutal effect of rationing by affordability is measured in shortened lives, increased disability, and pain. Is this what is medically necessary for people without insurance coverage? When each insurer cares only for its own covered population, care is fragmented, the whole is ignored, and the health status of Americans is poorer than that of the citizens of other industrialized countries.

THE RELATIONSHIP BETWEEN UTILIZATION AND QUALITY

Even if costs were not an issue, more would not necessarily be better. Too much care is as harmful as too little or the wrong kinds of care. There is a direct relationship between health care utilization and quality of care. The Institute of Medicine's National Roundtable on Health Care Quality classifies quality problems into three categories: overuse, underuse, and misuse.[26] In each category, the patient is unnecessarily exposed to serious risk and harm that can be measured in terms of lost lives, reduced functional status, and wasted resources.

Overuse occurs when the care's potential for harm exceeds its potential for benefit. Prescribing antibiotics for a simple cold and performing unnecessary hysterectomies are common examples of overuse. Misuse occurs when a preventable complication occurs although the right care was prescribed. For example, twice as many people die annually from medication errors as from motor vehicle accidents or breast cancer. Medication errors account for 44,000–98,000 deaths and cost $17 billion to $29 billion annually, according to the Institute of Medicine. Underuse is failing to provide care when it would have had a favorable outcome. Undetected and untreated hypertension and depression, failure to provide preventive care, and delayed palliative care typify significant underuse problems. According to National Roundtable data, these quality problems are similar in managed care and fee-for-service settings.[27]

IN SEARCH OF BALANCE

Because of the relationship between utilization and quality, researchers posit that for each disease or medical condition there is a quantitative relationship between the type of care provided, or *utilization*, and its benefit to the patient. In other words, benefit is a function of utilization. When the benefit is high, quality is high.

If the units of care provided and benefits were graphed, the data points would form a curve (see figure 5.3). Where the curve begins to crest is the point at which the patient receives the most benefit from the care provided. To the left of this point, the benefits are suboptimal because not enough units of care are provided. Across the crest of the curve, benefits stay constant despite additional units of care. The area to the right of the crest signifies deteriorating benefits due to excessive use of resources. In other words, resources are wasted and the patient is harmed. In theory, benefit-utilization curves prevent over- and underuse of scarce resources.

The problem is that the shapes of benefit-utilization curves are unknown. For these curves to be known, both units of care and benefits must be known for each medical condition. This information is unavailable despite the massive volumes of data health care annually collects. In fact, extensive research indicates a widespread variation in the ways diseases are diagnosed and treated.

For each medical condition, the type and the amount of care provided vary tremendously. Diagnostic and treatment decisions vary from region to region and from doctor to doctor. For instance, numerous studies substantiate significant geographical variation in the use of expensive procedures—such as hysterectomy, prostate surgery, and tonsillectomy—that do not result in better health status. These variations cannot be accounted for by clinical criteria or the severity of the patients' condition.[28]

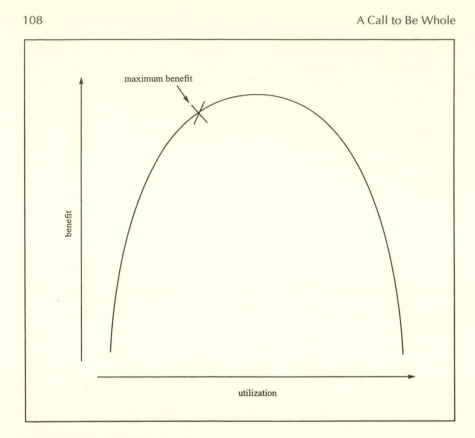

Figure 5.3 Benefit-Utilization Curve

Some physicians practice conservatively; others are quick to use the latest drug or diagnostic test. Despite claims that medicine is a scientific enterprise, a physician's clinical decisions are more dependent upon where the physician went to medical school, peer pressure, and information from trade associations than upon rigorous scientific evidence.

The vast majority of diseases do not have a single best treatment. For conditions, like chronic back pain, for which there is more than one recognized surgical treatment, there are also one or more equally feasible nonsurgical options. To further complicate matters, some conditions, such as simple high blood pressure, respond equally well or better to alternative modalities as they do to biomedicine's more costly and invasive pharmacopoeia.

In contrast to other industries, there is very little standardization in the delivery of medical care. Whether the procedure is as simple as the administration of antibiotics or as complex as coronary bypass surgery, the sequence of tasks, the types of equipment, the personnel, and the supplies used in these procedures vary significantly among institutions and even among physicians within one institution.

About 85 percent of all medical technology—medical devices, drugs, biologicals, and diagnostic and therapeutic procedures—commonly used by doctors and hospitals has never received any kind of rigorous scientific evaluation. Neither their true therapeutic benefits nor their cost benefits have been scientifically validated. Instead, their adoption is justified because of their "potential to benefit."[29]

Unfortunately, managed care acts as though benefit-utilization curves are known in its monitoring of physicians' clinical decisions and in its determination of covered benefits. On the utilization—or care—side of the equation, no one has yet constructed the databases to show which set of interventions is most likely to produce the best results, which providers are the most skillful, which hospitals do more of x procedure with fewer complications. Instead of basing their decisions on well-designed scientific research, most insurers' decisions regarding necessary care are made by their own technical review panels and are not subject to outside review.

Moreover, because we have conflated a modern concept of health with a postmodern concept of cure, the benefit side of the equation is equally confusing. On one hand, the term *benefit* refers to health outcomes, and *outcome* refers to the consequences of medical intervention. On the other hand, *benefit* refers to beneficiary and *beneficiary* refers to the recipient of care. Are we seeking what is beneficial for the nation's health, for the health of the individual, or for both? How can health care become more efficient, especially if the recipient lives in poverty or suffers from chronic or life-threatening sickness? Our answers to these questions depend upon whether we see the health care system through modern or postmodern eyes (see Table 5.3).

Table 5.3
Modern versus Postmodern Understanding of Health Care

Modern Understanding of Health Care	Post modern Understanding of Health Care
Based on Newtonian physics	Based on Einsteinian and quantum physics
Parts are primary.	Whole is primary.
Beneficiary of care is the individual patient.	Beneficiary of care is both the nation and the patient
Treatment is drugs and surgery to fix abnormal biomechanisms in the physical body.	A continuum of social and environmental interventions to promote population health including medical, behavioral, and spiritual interventions to promote personal health
Health outcomes are the function of physician competency.	Health is the outcome of the interaction of a continuum of determinants, only one of which is medical competency.

CAUGHT BETWEEN A MODERN AND A POSTMODERN UNDERSTANDING OF HEALTH CARE

Americans are caught between a rock and a hard place. If we hang on to the modern worldview, we lock ourselves into yesterday's thinking and perpetuate health care's vicious cycles. Able only to replicate what we already know, the best we can do is accelerate health care's inefficiencies: Costs increase while access and quality decrease.

Modernity posits that the material world is the only reality, perceives health care as an independent system, collapses all determinants of health to biological pathology, and reduces care to biomedical interventions that are instituted by providers, one patient at a time. Consequently, health is a commodity, and the conflict between utilization and benefit—between profit and care, in other words—is perceived as an individual problem, most visible in the context of the doctor-patient relationship, where cost-containment efforts have altered, if not eroded, the quality of care.

If we adopt the postmodern view, however, our behavior is driven from a radically different understanding. With this understanding, no thing is permanent; we and our systems are interrelated and interdependent; and what happens to any one part affects the whole. From this holistic view of people and their systems, health care is a social good, and cost, quality, and access are perceived as interdependent. In this light, rationing is a commitment to economic efficiency and to a predetermined level of care across a continuum of needs: preventive and acute, chronic, and life-threatening. In the best of all possible worlds, rationing strategies produce a health care system that is effective, efficient, and fair.

THE HEART OF HEALTH CARE REFORM

Ironically, the public's chief complaint—health care's soaring costs—is an obstacle to change. Health care is awash in money. One trillion dollars is a potent incentive for powerful interest groups to protect their economic benefits at weaker stakeholders' expense. On the other hand, a trillion dollars is enough for everyone if it's shared. How much is enough? is the heart of health care reform.

The dark underside of this question exposes us to our deepest fears—that there really are limits to life, to economic growth, and to the planet's resources. Also, any inquiry into enough challenges us to become real, or whole, to one another. This is another way of saying that making peace with life's limits largely depends on becoming more trusting and more trustworthy. The bright side, however, assumes abundance and interconnection: There is enough for everyone; it's safe to share.

DRAWING NEW BOUNDARIES, ADDING NEW FEEDBACK LOOPS

In systems language, sharing refers to rationing, which means not wasting resources. Rationing strategies mean adding novel feedback loops,

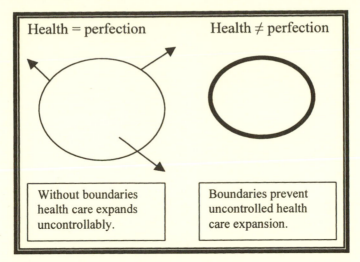

Figure 5.4 Boundaries Prevent Uncontrolled Growth

changing the flow of information and resources, and altering responsibilities. Sharing also means drawing new boundaries, adding new recipients, and evoking new values and meaning. No doubt some will receive fewer resources so that others can have more. Overall, sharing means a better-integrated, or healthier, health care system, and healthy systems are productive systems.

How much is enough? is a boundary issue. Boundaries by definition ration health care, for they determine the people and things that comprise the health care system. Drawing new boundaries means that we recognize that health care is not a panacea and that health is not a state of perfection: neither a state of complete physical, mental, and social well-being (the WHO definition) nor the absence of disease or injury (biomedicine's definition). Like infinity, perfection and panacea are all-encompassing, hence unbounded terms. Drawing new boundaries, we acknowledge that life and health and care have limitations (see figure 5.4).

Drawing new boundaries means engaging in new thinking. That is to say, we perceive health care not as an isolated system but as one system in a nested hierarchy of systems: the self, health care, our market economy, and an overarching worldview (see Figure 5.5). This holistic perspective reveals health care's true status as a part in a larger whole. It also reveals the root cause of escalating health care costs: The only connection now between health care and the market economy is a reinforcing feedback loop. Consequently, costs are destined to rise because the critical balancing loop is missing.

Sharing also signifies a global budget. Although the devil is in the details, global budgets alone don't tell us where the money will come from or how it will be spent. Someone still has to decide on price ceilings, expenditure caps, the determinants of health that belong to health care,

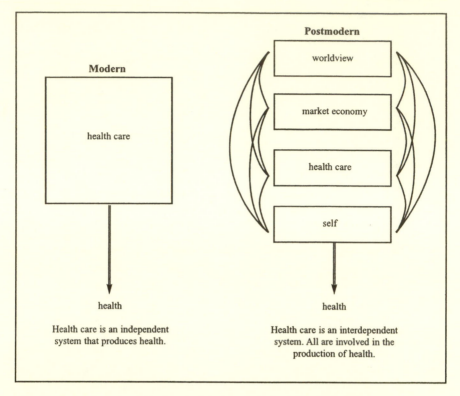

Figure 5.5 Modern versus Postmodern Perception of Health Care

and the types and distribution of services. Although price ceilings for
providers, payers, and purveyors and geographic distribution of services
are beyond the scope of this discussion, determinants of health that
belong to health care and types of services are relevant. They raise the
question, What is a standard benefits package, one that provides an adequate level of care?

DETERMINING THE RESOURCES IN A STANDARD
BENEFITS PACKAGE

The five determinants of health—societal, environmental, behavioral,
medical, and genetic—have both population and personal implications.
Societal and environmental determinants, which have a population effect
and belong to public health, are not part of a benefit package. However,
due to the growing concern that patients with chronic and life-threatening
conditions have different needs from those with acute conditions, there is
contentious debate regarding the medical and behavioral resources that
belong to an adequate benefit package. Here, behavioral resources include

supportive relationships and spiritual beliefs as well as coping and self-care skills.

Because the United States does not have a minimum standard level of covered benefits, the range of goods and services varies greatly for those with health insurance. Covered benefits vary according to carrier and type of plan. Generally, the more expensive the plan, the more comprehensive the benefits.

While health plans generally cover acute-care needs, most plans severely restrict mental health, home care, and rehabilitation services. Long-term care is distinct from acute care and must be purchased separately. Medicare and many other plans do not pay for prescription drugs, even though pharmaceuticals are the mainstay of biomedical care. For instance, chemotherapy, the mainstay of most cancer treatment, is not readily covered unless the plan includes pharmaceutical benefits. Coverage limitations are often not apparent until a person needs care. Then, it is too late to switch plans. Since the patient now has a preexisting condition, he or she risks being redlined or incurring more expensive premiums.

The Oregon Basic Health Services Program, commonly known as the Oregon Plan, is the most prominent attempt to determine a standard benefits package. Briefly, benefits are restricted to a list of 709 diagnosis-treatment pairs prioritized in order of health outcome. Funding priority is given to low-tech, inexpensive, preventive services that benefit many and to curative treatment for acute sicknesses. For example, prenatal care and immunizations receive high priority. Low priority is given to self-limiting conditions, such as a cold, and for conditions for which treatment is generally ineffective, such as surgery for lower back pain. Experimental procedures, such as bone marrow transplantation, are not funded at all. Successful in holding down costs while giving more poor people access to Medicaid benefits, the Oregon Plan is not perfect, but it's a good start.

Like other covered-benefits plans, the Oregon Plan is based on the modern understanding of health and disease. Treatment is limited to procedures that counteract flawed biology, all problems are treated as if they are acute, and patients are assumed to be uniform in their treatability. However, to continue to base an adequate level of care on collapsing chronic and life-threatening conditions to an acute production model is yesterday's thinking. In this era of chronic diseases, we still spend billions on high-tech cures and very little to relieve suffering and humanize care. Yet research shows that the medical, emotional, and functional outcomes of chronic illness depend upon supporting and strengthening the patients' capacity to manage their condition.[30] Similarly, it's been proven that the less-costly palliative and hospice care, whose outcome is death with dignity and comfort, better meets the needs of those with life-threatening illness.

Symptom relief is not enough for patients with chronic and life-threatening conditions. Health outcomes improve when care also includes self-management skills; adaptations for disabilities; advance care planning; caregiver and family support; and attention to grief, depression, and other emotional consequences of being sick. In short, an adequate level of care for these patients includes a continuum of care: medical care for symptom relief; other interventions that support and strengthen personal coping skills, health habits, and family and social relationships; and religious or spiritual beliefs.

Moreover, patients vary enormously. Especially within the categories of chronic and life-threatening sickness, the severity of the condition, the existence of other health problems, age, ability to follow a doctor's orders, availability of family and social support, and even the desire to live are not the same. In short, depending upon the constellation of physiological, psychological, and social variables, two patients with the same diagnosis may have radically different outcomes.

Although benefit-utilization curves can be calculated with mathematical precision, numbers all too neatly eclipse the human side of care. Because patients vary enormously, to what extent should an adequate level of care be malleable? For instance, should patients who are unable or unwilling to make lifestyle changes have the option of coronary bypass surgery or angioplasty if those lifestyle changes are mathematically more cost-effective but require impossible family adjustments? Should patients receive normally beneficial procedures that are likely to fail due to the patients' physical status? In other words, should the frail elderly receive kidney dialysis, a person with end-stage Lou Gehrig's disease be put on a ventilator, or should our young mom with cancer receive intensive treatment that might buy her a little more time?

Some degree of individualization is inevitable, so who has the authority to make allocation decisions? Should physicians have the authority to make resource allocation decisions because they understand the complexity of the patient's clinical condition and the typical outcome? Should insurers decide, managing care by micromanaging physicians? Or should the patients decide, since they are the ones who experience the consequences of the sickness and best know the value they place on aggressive or conservative care?

Although benefit-utilization curves have yet to be calculated for each type of resource and medical condition, we do know enough to allocate resources across the continuum of needs: prevention and acute, chronic, and life-threatening conditions. We also know that universal access, or an adequate level of care for all Americans, is salutary. Universal access allows those who don't now have health insurance access to medical care; eliminates the risk of losing health benefits because of a change in address, employment, age, or health status; and eliminates the devastation of losing health benefits when one loses one's job—a stressful time that often compromises health. Moreover, an adequate level of care for all Americans assures continuity of care—an issue of immense concern to people with serious illnesses, now frequently forced to find new providers and/or health plans after their payer dropped them.

SELF-ADVOCACY

Essentially, the economic reform of the 1980s turned health care into a commodity and the patient into a consumer. Today, shopping for health care is like shopping for a car or buying toothpaste; it exemplifies the need to let the buyer beware. No longer can insured patients assume the role of passive recipients of care, expecting their doctor to provide everything that might have potential benefit. As managed care has made explicitly clear, the doctor cannot give away that which does not belong to him or to her. No longer is the physician the advocate for the patient. Instead, with managed care, physicians must balance their own economic needs with the medical needs of the patient and with the economic needs of the payer.

Managed care presents the patient as a consumer. Instead of expecting his doctor to shop for him with a blank check, the patient is expected to be an informed consumer. To get the most for her dollar presupposes that the patient has some knowledge about the workings of her own body, some definition of health, and a familiarity with the different types of care. Generally speaking, patients inform themselves by reading what is written in medical journals, the popular press, and on the Internet; by talking with other patients about their experiences; and by relying on their doctors' clinical expertise.

Being an informed consumer not only obliges patients to understand their health plan but it requires them to know what they can afford. It means having some idea of what they consider the best buy for their money, even if that means choosing between their physical and their economic health. In other words, given the dynamics of the current system, the effective use of scarce resources is an individual affair. Rationing is occurring, but without the protection of a global budget and access to an adequate level of care.

Generally speaking, patients who get the best care are advocates for themselves and have thought about the questions What is health? What is care? and How much is enough? Self-advocacy does not mean being the expert or taking an adversarial stance against the system. Self-advocacy refers to speaking up for one's own goals and needs and being an active, decision-making agent in the delivery of one's care. There is enough latitude in the contemporary health care system for individuals to take more control over their own health than they usually assume. For example, about a third of the U.S. public shops outside the system, choosing alternative care to either supplement or supplant traditional health care.

At a minimum, the prerequisites to good decision making include: adequate information; appropriate identification of alternatives; a willingness to shape and be shaped by sickness; and condition-appropriate roles, goals, and values.

Adequate information means knowing what resources are available. On one hand, this includes knowing the specifics of one's health plan, which means keeping abreast of the plan's often-changing rules, benefits, and annual and lifetime limits; knowing one's rights and assigned responsibilities; and understanding the financial incentives the plan offers its physicians,[31] since how one's doctor is paid sometimes affects the amount and type of care received. On the other hand, adequate information means knowing how to maximize the time spent with the doctor, knowing when the needed care is more complex than the primary care physician can deliver, and how to demand to see a specialist, and knowing how to insist on receiving reasonable screening tests and other preventive care.

Appropriate identification of alternatives includes knowing which conditions are self-limiting and can safely be treated with home remedies, and knowing when body work, Ayurvedic medicine, acupuncture, or other alternative forms of care—either alone or in combination with health care—are the wisest use of scarce resources. It also means knowing how to gain the support and skills to manage chronic diseases and knowing which intervention is best for you, since the vast majority of diseases do not have one best treatment.

For instance, bypass surgery, angioplasty, and medical therapy are the choices for treatment of coronary heart disease, and each has different outcomes, risks, side effects, and costs. Symptom relief tends to be slower with medical management, although the risk associated with drug therapy is much smaller. Bypass surgery costs about $30,000, and about half of grafts clog within five years; 30–40 percent of angioplasties, which cost about $10,000 each, need to be redone within four to six months; and the typical medical therapy of beta-blockers, nitroglycerine, and cholesterol-lowering drugs costs about $3,500 annually. Despite the variation in risks and costs, five-year survival rates for angioplasty and bypass surgery are no better than the rates for those who are medically treated. In contrast, recent research has shown that coronary heart disease can be reversed without the use of drugs or surgery.[32] Blood flow to the heart is significantly improved with a constellation of lifestyle changes. Because coronary arteries actually become less blocked, the five-year survival rate is better. Although essentially free of side effects, lifestyle changes are not without costs. Old habits are hard to break; lifestyle changes aren't a magic bullet and don't have the glamour of technology. Also, the patient still needs to be monitored by a provider, and most payers do not cover this type of therapy.

Because not everything can be cured, patients either implicitly or explicitly decide how they will shape and be shaped by prolonged and progressing sickness. There is a complicated and reciprocal relationship between a person's biology and his biography. His roles, values, and goals define him as a person, locate him in the web of family and civic responsibilities, and shape his understanding of his sickness. However, roles, goals, and values often unravel when people get sick, and their disruption tends to make the sickness worse. Because it adds to the uncertainty in the practice of medicine, this reciprocal relationship makes medicine an art as well as a science. Informed patients, therefore, know what the doctor can and cannot do, and what changes they must make in themselves and what things they must learn to accept.

Paradoxically, self-advocacy does not mean that the patient needs her physician less. She will always depend upon her physician's clinical skills, expert knowledge, and experience. It does mean that the physician is drawn into the unquantifiable psychocultural world of the patient, and that the patient is drawn into an equally uncertain world of clinical decisions.

SELF-ADVOCACY IS NOT ENOUGH

Whether we use the term *shared decision making* or *self-advocacy* to describe the process of including patients in decision-making processes, both terms conceal as much as they reveal. The way health care is now organized, physicians and managed care function as the dominant decision-making agents for the patient. Yet neither group has adequately separated its own financial welfare from the patient's well-being. Moreover, employers and the government are the primary purchasers of health insurance. Although self-advocacy definitely helps the patient get the most for his or her health care dollar, individuals don't have sufficient clout to balance the payers' and providers' well-financed and politically connected trade and professional organizations. In short, the information flow is a one-way street, and patients as a stakeholder group are simply out of the loop.

Similarly, the term *self-advocacy* also reinforces the modern structure of health care and modernity's values: unlimited economic growth and perfect health. Both allow special interest groups to play on people's fears of explicit health care rationing. The word *self* here implies that health and access to care are personal concerns and perpetuates the stakeholder game of economic musical chairs. In such a context, self-advocacy readily slips into selfishness, and efficiency slips through our hands.

Postmodernity posits that large systems emerge from human thought and are animated by human hands, however. As postmodernity posits interconnectedness, self-advocacy refers to having a concern for the whole and, thereby, asserting as an individual health care's need for a global budget and that those in need have the right to an adequate level of care.

In this holistic context self-advocacy is not a selfish but a selfless state, because we go beyond the small, automatic-pilot version of ourselves. More mindful, we see that it is not efficient to shift costs and that without a global budget what one stakeholder debits as waste another stakeholder credits as profit. Because we are more mindful, our behavior changes, taking health care with us beyond its present vicious-cycle state.

QUESTIONS FOR THE READER

1. Is the purpose of health care to produce productive citizens? Is it a commodity to be sold to those who can afford its escalating price? Is it a social good available to all in need?

2. Most Americans have a laundry list of services or conditions that should or should not be covered. For instance, hospitalization; physician services; prenatal care; preventive services; drugs; and dental, vision, and nursing-home care are favorite items; plastic surgery, organ transplantation, and long-term ventilator or nutritional support for patients in a persistent vegetative state are typically excluded. What is on your list?

3. Knowing that health care can neither cure nor prevent chronic disease, aging, and disability, what is the role of traditional health care? What is the right distribution of resources among prevention and acute, chronic, and life-threatening care?

4. Where should the resources for custodial care (i.e., nursing-home care) come from?

5. Should alternative forms of care be covered?

6. How much are you willing to pay for health care? What benefits are important to you?

7. Should every business provide health insurance for its employees? How should the uninsured be covered?

8. If the United States adopts a global budget for health care, where should the monies come from? Payroll taxes? Corporate taxes? Other?

9. Should there be price ceilings on health care goods and services, such as physicians' and others' salaries, pharmaceutical goods, and other supplies?

10. Should there be expenditure caps on health care goods and services? How should these services be distributed?

11. If you were chronically ill, would you engage in an endless quest for a technological cure, or would you look to other resources to help you adapt to your sickness? Should chronic care include interventions that strengthen and support self-management skills, family and caregiver relationships, and spiritual beliefs?

12. As you age, will you chase after face-lifts and other scientific promises to keep yourself youthful? When you become so frail in body or mind that you can no

longer care for yourself, who do you expect to take care of you? What resources might be needed? Who will pay for your care?

13. What do you know about your health plan? What resources are available to you? Is it adequate to cover your needs?

14. What have you said to your family regarding goals and the types of care you expect if you experience a severe accident or a life-threatening illness? Does your physician know your expectations? Are your wishes formalized in a living will or in advanced directives?

15. If others' well-being demands any redistribution of your wealth, privileges, or prestige, what are you willing to share?

16. Do you want the same for others as you want for yourself? If not, why not?

17. Review your answers for the questions What is care? and What is health? If any of those answers conflict with your answers to How much is enough? change your answers until they are congruent.

18. What is the purpose of health care? Would your answers regarding the distribution of resources generate a health care system that is efficient, effective, and fair?

19. How would a global budget or a national health care system effect you? What impact would it have on each of the other stakeholder groups?

CHAPTER 6

Who Is Responsible?

All of us have to be for everybody. What the individual does first is to
have the integrity of handling the truth.

Buckminster Fuller

Words create pictures in our heads and stir up feelings. The word *responsibility* evokes images regarding leadership and power and stirs up issues of
roles and status. *Responsibility*, according to Webster's dictionary, means
being able to answer. Being able to answer tacitly implies the possession of
sufficient knowledge, authority, and resources to respond.

Responsibility has both a personal and a systems dimension. Persons
are autonomous agents; they manifest themselves in doing. Because
everything that we do begins as some kind of thought, and because
human beings and their systems are mutually enfolded, our inquiry into
responsibility also seeks to discover the influences that worldview and the
health care system have in shaping a person's behavior.

In systems language, when we ask, Who is responsible for the production of health? we are asking about socially sanctioned roles. We are asking about the capacity of those roles. On one hand, we are inquiring into
the authority, competencies (knowledge, behavior, and attitudes), and
privileges associated with roles that belong to health care. On the other
hand, we are also inquiring into access to resources involved in healing.
From a resource perspective, the question Who is responsible? is an
inquiry into the role society has authorized as having access to the
resources used in the production of health.

From Flood's perspective, however, Who is responsible? is an inquiry
into who possesses the knowledge power. Knowledge power is the notion

that "people in positions of power determine what is considered to be valid knowledge and consequently valid action."[1] Examining health care through the facet of knowledge power illuminates the fairness of the system's design. We see who is included, who is excluded, and the reasons why. In Flood's words, we see "who benefits from the efficiency of the process and the effectiveness of the structure."[2]

PHYSICIANS ARE RESPONSIBLE FOR PRODUCING HEALTH

In any health care system, the responsibilities of the patient and the healer are tacitly embedded in society's definition of health and are based on a worldview that is compatible with society's view of the human body. Like all constructs of human thought, these responsibilities are fluid, conforming to the container of their time. Before spirit was separated from matter and Isaac Newton explained the universe as a mechanical clock, knowledge power was the divine right of priests and kings. Then, the authority to heal belonged to priests, a responsibility that lasted until the power of prayer and the thirteenth-century church failed to stop the plague. Signaling a shift in power, the church's failure opened the door to the power of expert knowledge and the rise of modern science.

Our anatomically based health care system emerged from and is firmly grounded in the modern worldview wherein life is reduced to the laws of nature and the body is perceived as a mechanical entity with interchangeable parts. According to this linear, mechanical production model, health is something physicians produce.

Physicians fought hard for this responsibility, consolidating their knowledge power through the imposition of educational requirements and licensing laws and gaining sovereignty through third-party reimbursement and the marriage of science and technology. Perceived as scientists with stethoscopes, physicians by virtue of their training and medical license are the sole proprietors of the knowledge and skill necessary to make an objective, scientifically accurate diagnosis and to treat disease, or counteract its symptoms, with drugs or surgery. Their expert knowledge made them the agents responsible for the production of health. By 1930, the care of the sick had firmly become the medical profession's responsibility.

In the biomedical model, physicians have the authority to legitimize who is well and who is sick, which makes physicians gatekeepers to economic and social benefits as well as to health care's services. The doctor-patient relationship is supported by an expensive array of biotechnology that is paid for by third-party payers; physicians, vested with the authority to make life-and-death decisions, assume a kind of paternalistic responsibility for their patients. In this traditional relationship, the patients' limited role was to seek competent treatment and follow the doctors' orders.

TALCOTT PARSONS'S SICK ROLE

Every society ascribes a moral value to sickness. This cultural variable delineates the particular benefits, obligations, and stigmas associated with being sick. The sick role is always a socially institutionalized role, and biomedicine has institutionalized what is known as Parsons's sick role.[3] Talcott Parsons was an American sociologist who saw sickness as a kind of social deviancy that needed to be controlled; otherwise, it would spread like a contagious disease among susceptible members of the population.

According to Parsons, sickness is the loss of capacity to perform one's socially expected tasks or social roles. The sick role posits that sick people are not culpable for becoming sick, that they are entitled to care, and that they can expect to be relieved of their usual family, civic, and economic responsibilities. In return for these benefits, they are obligated to seek *technically* competent care, be motivated to get well, and do everything possible to get well. Conceptually, the sick role was designed to protect society as much as the individual. Although the role conditionally legitimizes sickness, it comes at a price.

Sickness is stigmatized; being sick is deviant behavior. Dependency and compliance are the coin for protection and care. Even though society mobilizes the community's resources to help the sick individual, mobilization is done not because it is the humane thing to do but to reaffirm the productive value of health. Making patients dependent on the physician to legitimize their status and allow access to society's resources, Parsons posited, would both proscribe using sickness as method to dodge civic responsibilities and facilitate the patient's recovery.

Parsons was among the first sociologists to see the doctor-patient relationship as a dyad with reciprocal responsibilities. The physician, by virtue of his training and licensure laws, is the sole proprietor of the necessary competencies for healing. The physician is guided not by self-interest but by altruism and is expected to restore health to the patient, whatever the sacrifice or cost to the physician, the patient, or society.

Although the physician is expected to act in the best interest of the patient, the physician is also an agent for social control. Because of the perception that scientific evidence is objective, or morally neutral, society has given the physician the authority to legitimize who is sick and the authority to use the community's resources on the patient's behalf. This makes the physician a gatekeeper. Today, physicians have a say in who can drive a car, get a job, stay home from work, qualify for disability benefits, go to summer camp, and get married. Likewise, physicians have a say in deciding who is competent to stand trial, who is likely to be dangerous to himself or others, and who is too incompetent to manage her own affairs.

Reciprocally, patients are those who the doctor attests as being sick; that is, they have a demonstrable biological pathology. Thus they can expect access to care and to be excused from their usual responsibilities. However, if the patient is not sick in the correct way, he is a hypochondriac; if she seems to be taking financial or other advantage of being sick, she's a malinger; and he's labeled neurotic if he doesn't get well. Any one of these conditions can disqualify the patient from access to society's resources. Consequently, the reciprocal role responsibilities inherently produce a childlike patient and a paternalistic physician.

WORKERS' COMPENSATION

Workers' compensation is the hallmark application of the sick role. A benefit awarded to workers whose sicknesses are work related, workers' compensation entitles the employee to financial coverage for the medical care of work-related disorders and to partial income replacement while he or she is unable to work. Briefly, the workers' compensation system is a trade-off: Workers give up their right to sue for negligence, and employers assume liability for work-related disorders. Based on the assumption that physicians can distinguish between injuries and sickness caused by employment and those that are not, society has made physicians the gatekeepers to these resources.

Ideally, workers' compensation is designed to help the employer and the employee achieve the same thing: the ability to be productive. The employee wants to earn a living, and employers want productive employees. Both groups have incentives to maintain their part of the bargain. Partial income replacement and appropriate medical expenses are incentives for employees to get well and quickly return to work. Similarly, having a healthy workforce and a work environment reasonably free of health hazards was considered a better bargain to employers than paying the costs of work-related disorders. In actuality, the system is far from ideal. The incentives no longer seem to work, and physicians are in the difficult position of choosing between the employer's economic interests and the employee's welfare.

The gatekeeper function is predicated on the assumption that medical determinations are scientific, objective, and impersonal. The physician is expected to determine occupational causality, and the physician is also expected to care for the patient. In actuality, neither action is value-neutral. If the disorder is determined not to be work related, the physician's decision benefits the employer. If the disorder is determined to be work related, the employee benefits. Despite the putative objectivity of the physician, the effect of social forces upon the recognition of occupational disorders, the presence of management, the influence of economic forces, and the physician's feelings for the patient affect his or her decisions as much as or more than the medical data.

By definition, occupational disorders are due to causal factors, such as unsafe conditions or hazardous substances in the work environment. Theoretically, there is a straight line between cause and effect. An errant saw results in a carpenter with a gashed thumb, for example. For many occupational disorders, however, cause and effect is not so clear-cut. Many of them have long induction periods; for instance, lung cancer in uranium miners. Some disorders also involve multiple causative agents; for example, cigarette smoking increases the risk of lung cancer in uranium miners. Still other disorders, such as lower back pain, have an indistinct relationship to work.

While the workers' compensation system works reasonably well with straightforward, nominally expensive claims, multifactorial causation introduces considerable uncertainty into the physician's determination of the specific relative contribution of occupational and non-work-related causes of disease. For complaints that do not have a distinct etiology, there is frequently a wide range of competing but scientifically justifiable opinion about occupational origins of a claim. Generally, as in the case of lung cancer that flight attendants attributed to secondhand smoke or hand and wrist disorders in meat cutters, determinations tend to be made as a result of class action suits rather than by medical data. Moreover, tort determinations typically occur after the media has brought the disorder to the public's attention.

Roughly a $55 billion industry, paid for by the employer and providing health care and income to disabled and injured workers, workers' compensation is second in size to Social Security Disability Insurance.[4] Even though the physician is allegedly neutral, the physician has obligations to the employer and/or insurance carrier that pays him or her, as well as to the patient. No one can serve two masters well, so the question is, who is the physician responsible to care for: the patient, the employer, or the payer?

In short, workers' compensation puts physicians in a double bind. In keeping with biomedicine's concern for the prevention and cure of disease, physicians have tacitly assumed responsibility for the healthiness and safety of the work environment. The syllogism is, if biomedicine does *not* determine the disorder to be work related, then the environment must be essentially free of harmful agents. This logic is flawed, however. For starters, scientific evidence is not neutral but is always socially mediated. Moreover, there is not a direct causal relationship, or a linear relationship, between nondetermination and a safe, hazard-free work environment.

In other words, the fact that the employee can't prove that the work environment caused his or her health problem doesn't mean that the work environment is safe and hazard-free. In fact, there is reliable documentation that corporate management permits worker exposure to potent carcinogens until the death rate can no longer be ignored,[5] that employers are increasingly casting safety policies in economic rather than human terms,[6] and that employers are using the courts to appeal and delay the implementation of health and safety procedures.[7]

Moreover, the function of biomedicine is to treat individual patients, one body at a time. It is not the purpose of biomedicine to intervene upstream, for the important nonmedical resources—the regulation, surveillance, and control of the persons and groups that inform social relationships—are beyond a physician's control. Products, production methods, production rates, staffing, and the context of the employer-employee relationship are outside the physician's authority, controlled by the employer and the state.

The best the physician can do is reframe the problem to express the disorder in a language that makes it appear to be part of one individual's physical world, eclipsing the social determinants of health and neutralizing management's responsibilities. For instance, workers complaining of physical fatigue and mental fatigue—generated by shift work, downsizing, understaffing, fast-paced working conditions, and rapidly changing technology—are typically treated with antidepressant drugs or told to attend stress-management classes. Similarly, the 5.6 percent rise in death from heart attack and the 3.1 percent rise in death from stroke that occur with a 1 percent rise in unemployment[8] are *not* considered to be work related because the individuals were not employed at the time of death.

Although physicians have fought for—and have been handsomely rewarded for—the gatekeeper role, assuming responsibility for the care of sick or injured employees is one thing. But tacitly assuming responsibility for the healthiness of the work environment is a responsibility that physicians can neither logically nor ethically assume. By perpetuating the belief that biomedicine is responsible for the healthiness of the workplace, biomedicine both conceals the employer and government incentives and sanctions that reward the retention of workplace hazards and foster health-denying behavior and tacitly enables government and corporate leaders to ignore their responsibilities to the health of the workforce.

Although medical knowledge is needed and is vital to ensuring a safe and healthy workforce, corporate and political leaders also have responsibilities to health. In truth, their actions affect the health of whole populations, for the sphere of influence of corporate and political leaders is much larger than that of individual physicians. In thinking about how to resolve this dilemma, Allard Dembe acknowledges that workers—like other members of society—need access to prompt, effective health care, income replacement for work incapacity, and protection against environmental health hazards:

Removing the need for physicians to make individual judgments as to whether particular patients are suffering from "occupational diseases" does not necessarily imply that enforcement of safety and health in the work place will become any less aggressive. On the contrary, if an insurance and health care system provide quality care and income replacement to patients irrespective of occupational etiology, then it would be more important than ever to ensure that the penalties and enforcement activities of the governmental safety and health agencies are strong and effective.[9]

THE STIGMA OF BEING SICK

In theory, the sick role protects access to care. People who can't care for themselves are not abandoned but are cared for by other members of society. In practice, however, society is only intermittently dutiful. Because the benefits, obligations, and stigmas of the sick role are actually quite labile, the sick are often shunned, blamed, or discounted. Access to health care's resources is also variable, influenced by some combination of disease, gender, ethnicity, politics, financial incentives, and the mass media.

The more that disease is considered socially or morally wrong, the more the afflicted person seems to be culpable, and the more threatening disease is to society, the more likely the patient will be stigmatized. For example, the public sentiment toward people with heart disease or breast cancer is in direct contrast to public sentiment toward those infected with HIV. Similarly, considerable evidence shows that the lower the family's income, the less likely the person is to have access to sick role benefits.

Mental illness tends to be more stigmatized than physical illness, and incurable sicknesses are more stigmatized than acute afflictions. Women's health problems are more likely to be discounted than men's because women continue to be stereotyped as nervous, irritable, and prone to hysteria. The health problems of low-wage earners, the marginally productive, and the disenfranchised are more likely to be discounted than those of their more fortunate neighbors. Finally, if an affliction is chronic or associated with lifestyle, the afflicted person is more likely to be blamed. For example, poor personal health habits are blamed for the plague of heart disease affecting most of Appalachia,[10] but the region's poverty, social isolation, and environmental pollution are not taken into account.

Having political, economic, and social overtones, stigmas tend to be associated with diseases—such as AIDS and leprosy—that are largely endemic, have a long incubation period, are seemingly incurable, are disfiguring and progressively crippling, are associated with low standards of living, or have the potential to overwhelm society's economic resources and medical facilities.[11]

In theory, the sick person is not culpable, but victim blaming is an American habit. Across the broad provider-payer-policy continuum there is evidence that the chronically ill, those in need of long-term rehabilitation, and the disabled are stigmatized, and subtle imputations of culpability drive a wedge between the healthy and the sick. At the least, the stigmatized are deprived of compassion; at the worst, they are denied their claim to health care's resources.

BLAME AND COUNTERBLAME

It's an American habit to ask Who is responsible? That, as everyone knows, means Who is to blame? Blame is the shadow side of responsibility, and Americans have expensively incorporated blame into Parsons's sick role. If the patient fails to get well, the patient is deviant or the doctor is incompetent. Either way, economic and emotional consequences befall whomever is culpable.

The patient risks being fired from the doctor's care and losing the benefits associated with the sick role, such as having access to a specialist, or qualifying for workers' compensation benefits if the affliction is work related. Reciprocally, the physician risks being perceived as incompetent and incurring financial penalties imposed by managed care. To avoid financial penalties, many physicians take a proactive stance and deselect patients who have histories of high costs, poor compliance with treatment regimens, or a poor response to treatment.[12]

Patients who evoke feelings of failure in their physicians are often labeled bad. Typically, bad patients are those who complain of ever-new symptoms or are hard to diagnose; are angry, demanding, or ungrateful; are dirty or hard to understand; or are obese, smoke, or are otherwise perceived as culpable. Thus, if the patient is not sick in the correct way, he or she is usually perceived a hypochondriac, a malingerer, or a neurotic. Any one of these conditions can disqualify the patient from access to care.

Difficult-to-treat patients are often referred from provider to provider. Each provider, in turn, tries to fix the problem, feels a sense of failure, and, finally, displaces the responsibility for failure on the patient. By firing the patient from his or her care, the physician is freed from emotional and economic liabilities.

In contrast, good patients are those who are grateful and who cause the physician to feel in control and competent in the fight against death and disease. Good patients don't take up much time, have legitimate diseases, unquestioningly submit to technological interventions, respond quickly to efforts to alleviate their symptoms, and comply with the doctor's orders. Similarly, the competent physician is swift, decisive, and objective; reduces problems to a malfunctioning body part; and aggressively uses technology to bring the body's biology under control.

Economics aside, blame and counterblame arise largely because modernity presents disease as a molecular problem. Unfortunately, this discounts the mystery of life and leads to the overestimation of physicians' technical competency. It also discounts the effect the severity of disease, preexisting conditions, the patient's home life, and the patient's beliefs and values regarding health have on the probability of the patient getting well.

Human beings are highly complex, a physical, psychological, social, and spiritual ensemble. Still, we act in accordance with modernity's linear model and hold patients and physicians responsible. We assume that if a patient would only comply with a competent doctor's orders, the outcome of medical interventions could be determined with the certainty of a chemical reaction in an Ehrlenmeyer flask.

THE COMPROMISED THERAPEUTIC RELATIONSHIP

Unfortunately, biomedicine's modern, materialistic, reductionistic concepts have brought us to another postmodern dilemma. The sick and their physicians are trapped between two evils if perfect health is not restored: the stigma of deviancy and the stigma of incompetency. This is another way of saying that trying harder won't make doctors more competent or patients more compliant.

When the physician is perceived as superior, or an expert, and the patient is perceived as a biological problem, neither the patient nor the physician can afford, in Becker's terms, to be *real* to each other. In short, each protects the integrity of his or her role by objectifying the other.

Physicians are perceived as the ones in control, yet, paradoxically, the physician's own history and his or her fullness as a physical, psychological, social, and spiritual being are eclipsed by his or her technical expertise. Furthermore, to avoid becoming too emotionally involved with their patients, physicians maintain a professional distance. Because the relationship is literally mechanical, it follows that the patient, then, is unaware of the physician's own fears and frustration with the limits of time, resources, and human finitude. Or the patient may engage in self-protective behavior and discount the physician's own history and human limitations. The physician doesn't feel cared for; his or her competency is threatened.

If the physician feels his competency is threatened, a typical response is to label the patient deviant. Patients sense this label, for the physician's behavior is abrupt and discourteous. Aware that he has to wait longer than others, that her complaints are discounted and her concerns are ignored, patients do not feel cared for. Devoid of comfort, kindness and advice, the relationship is empty. In self-defense, the patient blames the doctor for being incompetent. Patients who need to prove this point sue their physicians for malpractice. Ironically, patients who don't feel cared for are more likely to sue than are those whose care was technically compromised but who are satisfied with the therapeutic relationship.

Because old age, chronic conditions, and life-threatening illness can't be cured, modern beliefs place responsibilities on doctors and patients that neither can fulfill. These conditions *can* be cared for, however. The problem is that the old belief that organizes the structure of health care gets in the way: Medical technology is the only valid form of care.

Health care has yet to move from its mechanistic perception of the physical body to a postmodern understanding of health. Medical knowledge and resources are still based on the care of acute conditions for which the full clinical course spans a few days or weeks, and the patient's role is largely passive. Because the patient's condition is reduced to a biological problem and because the curative belief is ever present, roles are structured so that neither patients nor physicians have access to low-tech resources or have the mutual support necessary to be satisfied with anything less than perfection.

CARE IS MUTUAL IN A HEALTHY RELATIONSHIP

Biomedicine can't help people learn to discover their wholeness in the face of diminished physiology. As Arthur Frank states, people aren't asked, What do you wish to become in this experience? How will you shape your illness and be shaped by your illness? or How will this guide you in future decisions?[13]

Patients who are more autonomous do find a way to articulate their feelings. Receiving comfort and support to adapt to their limitations, these patients eventually find a new identity and add new meaning to their lives. Moreover, they suffer less than patients who behave as though technology will restore them to their former selves, saving them from having to adapt to a new way of being.

When the relationship is reciprocally rich in information, the physician is drawn into the unquantifiable psychosocial and spiritual world of the patient, and the patient is drawn into an equally uncertain world of clinical decisions. Paradoxically, limits are acknowledged, although neither party has to hide the fullness of who he or she is to fit the other's image. In this moment, each cares for the other.

This world of uncertainty offers benefits to both patients and providers. When treatment springs from mutual respect and reciprocal responsibility, trust is deepened, and informed consent is more informed. Having laid their cards on the table, both know with greater clarity what is at stake, responsibilities are balanced, care is reciprocal, and blame and counterblame are laid aside.

Still the patient's advocate, the physician gives what is his or hers to give: skill, knowledge, diligence, and advice. Through the physician's guidance, the patient better understands what he or she must do alone, what the doctor can and cannot do.

The patient is not a passive recipient. Knowing what can be cured and what must be managed; the probable risks and gains; that technology has side effects; and the costs to the body, the psyche, and the pocketbook, the patient accepts the trade-offs. When the outcome is generally what both expect, mutual feelings of competency and faith in the efficacy of the clinical decisions pervade the doctor-patient relationship.

DYSFUNCTIONAL SYSTEM ↔ DYSFUNCTIONAL ROLES

Responsibility means the ability to answer, or respond. From a systems perspective, the dysfunctional doctor-patient relationship is a symptom of a systems problem. Systems shape behavior; neither the physician nor the patient is truly an independent agent. A complex bureaucracy tightly controls the patient's access to care and increasingly controls the nature of doctor-patient interaction. For instance, there are volumes of rules, policies, and procedures affecting how physicians will be reimbursed, where they can practice, and which procedures they can perform.

Basically, blame and counterblame are painfully personal ways of saying that traditional roles are not effective. Less-personal evidence of role failure includes the rising numbers of malpractice lawsuits and the embrace of alternative medicine by patients and the rising rates of suicide, substance abuse, and early retirement of physicians.

Parsons did not invent the sick role; he reported what society had already constructed. Reinforced by our institutions, social roles don't exist independently from the worldview that infuses them. In other words, because modernity presents the universe as a mechanical clock, we should expect to see this notion repeated in our understanding of disease, in the responsibilities assigned to physicians, and in the organization of health care itself.

At the same time that medical doctors were using the scientific argument to garner power in the court of biomedicine, Frederick W. Taylor was establishing management as a science. The organization of work inside health care is very much based on Taylor's principles of scientific management, which, too, emerge from a mechanical-clock view of the world. Taylor's goal was to maximize profits by making work more efficient. Briefly, his principles include hierarchical control, clear lines of authority, the separation of planning and operations, and a division of labor with specialization and standardization of tasks.[14]

Health care is very much concerned with efficiency, and health care incorporates all of Taylor's principles. The mechanical nature of all health care relationships is clearly seen in the split between the delivery and the financing of care, and in the fragmented delivery of care. The patient's body belongs to the medical doctor, the patient's mind belongs to the psychiatrist, the chaplain is in charge of the patient's spirit, and the social worker is responsible for the social dimension of care. Even the role of the medical ethicist reflects Taylor's principles. Largely restricting their focus to "good" clinical decisions and the therapeutic benefit of medical technology, ethicists rarely get involved in other moral issues such as access to care or the morale of health care workers.

Having declared quantifiable data more real than subjective qualities, we have allowed these efficiencies to reduce human beings to objects used in the production of health and to economic statistics. Love and respect don't count. Moreover, we are caught in the trap of our own thinking. Insofar as health care is organized according to a worldview that understands people as machines, neither the patient, the physician, nor the insurance executive can perceive him- or herself as, or be perceived as, a moral agent.

In other words, working inside their professional boxes, keeping their professional distance, no one can be real, or whole. When the free and natural expression of thoughts and feelings is not permitted, people can't mutually care for one another. In short, the qualitative, or moral, aspect of the relationship is eclipsed by a mechanical structure. Using Wilber's language, there is no "We"; human relationships are organized as "I" and "It." Devoid of We, mechanical structures inherently breed discontent, distrust, and competition.

A systems perspective tells us that the role itself is more influential than the individual in the role. That is, roles in systems are like roles in a play. Richard Burton and Laurence Olivier may not play Hamlet the same way, but we'll always know they are playing Hamlet. The rights, privileges, and responsibilities belong to the social role, not to the individual. People are not independent agents but act largely in accordance with the social norms, policies, procedures, rules, values, and goals that inform their social role.

Although this information is personalized and translated into action, there's a rub. To understand health care's dysfunction we need to see more than personalities and events, but the mechanical nature of health care causes us to see personalities and events. However, seeing the constraints inherent in our roles frees us to behave in new, more healthy ways toward one another. Paradoxically, once we change, the structure of health care changes too.

RESPONSIBILITY INVOLVES ACCESS TO RESOURCES

Being responsible involves the ability to access resources and information important to the production of health. In this era of chronic diseases, health care spends billions treating one person at a time with high-tech cures. In 2000, chronic disease accounted for about 70 percent of all deaths and more than 60 percent of health care spending.[15] As the Institute of

Medicine has pointed out,[16] the delivery and financing of health care lag behind the needs of those with chronic diseases; those with life-threatening illness feel this lag as well.

Chronic health conditions—alcoholism, HIV, diabetes, congestive heart failure, Alzheimer's, and so forth—affect an estimated 100 million Americans. Chronic means that the person is sick but stable. As well as needing traditional medical care, patients with chronic conditions also need long-term monitoring and time-intensive clinical and behavioral interventions necessary to build the confidence and skills required for self-management and the prevention of complications.

Life-threatening conditions primarily effect the elderly, in that 70 percent of all deaths in the United States occur in people older than sixty-five.[17] *Life-threatening* means that the sick person is no longer stable but is frail and failing. Death may not be imminent, but the doctor wouldn't be surprised if the person died within a year. People with life-threatening conditions need pain and symptom management, help with hygiene and other activities of daily living, emotional and social support, and attention to spiritual needs. With the exception of hospice, which for a host of reasons serves only about 15 percent of the dying population, these services are not covered by third-party reimbursement.

The bulk of the day-to-day care of chronically ill patients and those with life-threatening disease falls upon the patient's families. Families bear a huge responsibility. As well as being the patient's advocate and helping the activities of daily living, the family also provides such things as emotional support, income replacement, housekeeping, grocery shopping, and transportation. The way health care is designed, it is easy for a ninety-year-old to get open-heart surgery, but it is almost impossible to get the soft-tech care vital to living with dignity and comfort while dying.

In effect, the family is an unpaid provider. The problem is, who is responsible for paying for these services if the family is unable to pay? All too often, families find themselves trapped between two bad choices. One is institutionalizing a sick child or divorcing a sick spouse in order to receive Medicaid; the other is draining the family physically, emotionally, and financially, and then being eligible for Medicaid.

Access to resources is a tremendous concern for those with chronic and life-threatening conditions. In acute conditions, outcomes largely depend on the competent use of drugs and surgery, and these 20 percent of the determinants of health are under the physicians' control and reimbursed by third-party payers. However, the resources that bring comfort and dignity to those with chronic and life-threatening conditions are not covered benefits. For example, physicians are not reimbursed for teaching and monitoring patients, for providing emotional support to patients and their families, for the planning of care and the coordination of multiple specialists and nonmedical caregivers, or for helping the family access appropriate community agencies. Typically too weak or ill informed to be his or her own advocate, or having a family that is too dysfunctional to help, the patient needs the physician's aid to access these nonmedical determinants of health. Yet providing them makes the physician less productive, for he or she is not reimbursed.

Pointing to the inadequacies in the acute-care model and stating that improvements can't be achieved by tampering with the existing system, the Institute of Medicine has described systemic changes needed for the effective management of chronic disease.[18] They include patient-centered care; inter-disciplinary terms; evidence-based decision making; new information systems designed for on-going clinical monitoring and sharing information among team mebers; freeing chronic care from the existing maze of regulations and reimbursement methods; and integrating the now-separate "unrelated management, information systems, payment mechanisms, financial incentives, and quality oversight for each segment of care. Others also recommend including incentives for proactive, continuous care."[19]

Although the needed systemic changes are well known, the wrong stakeholders are usually held accountable. Because the delivery and financing of health care are treated as separate functions, the public largely perceives providers as responsible for the production of health and the quality of care. Yet providers' hands are tied, as the provision of resources is largely in the payer's hands.

WHO IS RESPONSIBLE FOR THE POPULATION'S HEALTH?

In the biomedical model, physicians are responsible for the production of health; health is perceived as a state of complete physical, mental, and social well-being, not merely as the absence of disease; and the determinants of health are collapsed into medical technology and placed in the physicians' hands. This model, which emerges from the modern worldview and institutionalizes values compatible with our economic system, reinforces (1) a mechanical understanding of the body, (2) the assumption that health is an individual concern, and (3) the commodification of care.

By describing health as the absence of disease and by claiming responsibility for the prevention, as well as the cure of disease, physicians have implicitly assumed responsibility for the health of the population. This responsibility physicians can neither logically nor ethically carry.

Population health is influenced principally by the social and environmental determinants of health. These two determinants represent about 55 percent of the determinants of a population's health. In comparison, medical care represents about 20 percent; health behaviors, 20 percent; and genes and biology, the remaining 5 percent.

Controlling about 20 percent of the determinants of health, physicians at best can reduce what are actually social and environmental problems to molecular problems that appear in one patient's physical body. However, the mismatch of resources and responsibility is costly in terms of dollars and outcome. Americans spend 14 percent of the GDP on 20 percent of the determinants of health, and the health status of Americans ranks thirty-seventh in the world.

Unaware of the thought that is organizing health care, we tend to blame the victim for his or her poor health. Ironically, victim blaming is a way to block access to care and to shift costs back to patients. Economic sanctions on individuals, such as sin taxes on cigarettes and alcohol or high insurance premiums for those engaging in at-risk behaviors, are popular. At the policy level, however, the premise that chronic diseases can be prevented through positive health habits is a move toward cost containment and a retrenchment from the notion that health care is a right and the sick are entitled to care.

This is not to say that health habits do not make a difference—they do. Positive health behaviors are protective against disease and are significant to the management of chronic disease. However, to focus solely on an individual's poor health habits obscures the actual control the individual has regarding the safety of working conditions, the wages and benefits he or she is paid, or the safety of his or her neighborhood.

For example, at the low end of the economic continuum, 26 million Americans live below the federally defined poverty level, and 11 million of them receive no federal assistance.[20] To generalize, this income level doesn't support an adequate diet rich in fresh fruits and vegetables. Starches and fats are low-cost calories. Afraid to leave their house, people are sedentary, and to take the edge off their hunger, weariness, and fear, low-income people self-medicate with alcohol and tobacco. Another generalization is white-collar workers who complain of physical or mental fatigue due to shift work, downsizing, understaffing, fast-paced working conditions, and rapidly changing technology. These workers, who usually have health insurance, are typically treated with antidepressant drugs and told to attend a stress management class. The problem is, neither self-medication nor prescription drugs creates social capital, nor do they repair the fractured, fractious civic relationships that trigger the stress that triggers disease. Love, trust, and respect, the ingredients of healthy relationships, come from the heart.

Similarly, the incidence of teenage pregnancies, low-birth-weight infants, and infant mortality indicates how a population will fair later in life. Enormous amounts of data show the reciprocal relationships of childhood development, economic productivity, and adult health status. Simply put, nutritionists know that third-world villagers are physically smaller than Americans not because they are genetically destined to be small, but because their caloric intake is inadequate for growth. To add insult to injury, their small, underfed bodies prevent them from working enough to produce the food they need to grow bigger and stronger.

Children raised in emotional or economic poverty or in toxic environments are like these villagers; all are trapped in a vicious cycle of inadequate resources. While prenatal medical care is an important resource, other resources are more important, such as a living wage and decent affordable housing, flexible working hours, good childcare facilities, parenting skills, and good-quality public schools. These resources are certainly outside of health care's control.

Despite the success of the most savvy and determined patients in piecing health care's resources together for personal use, one successful patient doesn't affect the health of a population group. One person's positive health habits simply cannot mitigate the more powerful array of social and environmental determinants; one individual's sphere of influence is much too small to affect the health of many. Occasionally, a grassroots leader like Erin Brockovich or Lois Marie Gibbs—a resident of the infamous Love Canal who is known to many as the mother of the Superfund—stands up for herself and the health of her community. But such selfless advocacy is rare and very rarely is translated into national policy.

The irony is perverse: "Most resource investment is at the personal level and is inversely related to spheres of action most likely to have the largest impact on population health."[21] Downstream biomedical care intervention is not prevention. In caring for the health of the population, mammograms, bone density tests, and other types of screening can't hold a candle to the provision of jobs, a fair distribution of income, a safe environment, and a good quality of civic relationships. Policies, regulations, and surveillance mechanisms that govern the civic infrastructure and control production methods, employment relationships, and protect environmental safety are way beyond the physician's authority.

The problem is that the structure of health care, by placing responsibility for health in the hands of physicians, conceals responsibilities of corporate executives and government officials regarding the health of the population. It's unfair to blame the patient for poor health habits and expensive to expect health care to reverse upstream damage. Although it is tempting to blame physicians—for the knowledge, practice, and structure of biomedicine is largely the result of physicians' knowledge power—in actuality, the personal/population health dilemma is another example of dysfunctional roles and a dysfunctional system.

MANAGED CARE SHIFTS RESPONSIBILITIES

In 1951, when Parsons published the sick role, health care was neither an industrial complex nor a growth industry. Health care was more altruistic and less commercial. With technology in its infancy, the doctor had relatively little to offer the patient other than his or her own knowledge, experience, and effort. Then, too, private health insurance had just established itself as a customary employee benefit.

As we've seen, third-party, cost-plus reimbursement reinforced the growth of medical technology because third-party payers unquestionably covered the costs. In the third-party, cost-plus arrangement, the payer was simply a silent partner in the doctor-patient relationship. Knowledge power was largely in the hands of physicians. By the mid-1980s, however, escalating health care costs became a serious concern for employers and the government. Claiming it could control health care costs through aggressive contracting and utilization control, managed care rose to power, signifying the consolidation of knowledge power to the insurance section. That means fiduciary responsibilities now trump clinical responsibilities.

With managed care, the payer is no longer a silent partner in the doctor-patient dyad. Instead of assuming all of the financial risk, managed care has shifted a portion of it to the patient and the provider. The physician is no longer shopping for the patient with a blank check; with managed care the physician is also shopping with some of his or her own money.

The medical ethicist E. Haavi Morreim suggests that this new medical setting is forcing society to reconsider the reciprocal responsibilities within the doctor-patient dyad:

[T]he physician is not obligated to bypass legitimate contracts or program limits, to ignore other patient's competing interests, or even to efface totally his own interests. Rather the physician owes his patient what is his to give. He owes some very traditional duties, such as professional competence, compassion, and honesty. And he has some rather new duties, including economic advocacy, economic disclosure, and a close scrutiny of the economic structures and institutions with which he affiliates.

Conversely,...patients must assume a new role. Whereas we may be accustomed to thinking only about protecting the patient's freedom to choose as he wishes and act as he pleases, it is now time to expect the patient to exercise responsibility for his own choices not only over individual medical decisions, but also over other matters, such as lifestyle choices and selection of health care coverage. The patient's active participation in shaping the new economics of healthcare is not merely to be permitted; it is to be expected.[22]

While Morreim succinctly captures the new and reciprocal responsibilities managed care has injected into the doctor-patient dyad, Morreim's argument presupposes that the physician and the patient have the knowledge, the power, and the social support to make right and good decisions. In actuality, the power shift is fraught with hazards; the doctor and the patient are caught in situations in which the old rules no longer apply, but the new rules and responsibilities are far from clear.

For starters, patients have only limited authority to select their health plan, and therefore their physician. Employers pick the slate of plans, although employees can often choose between two or more plans. Searching for the least costly plan, employers may change the types and number of plans offered to employees annually. Insurance companies have adopted a one-year mentality, in part because employers are likely to change plans and in part to maximize their profits through annual changes in rules and covered benefits. Because each plan is a contract with a limited network of physicians and hospitals, and because these contracts, too, change frequently, a long-term patient-physician relationship and continuity of care are impossible.

Moreover, what *must* be covered varies from state to state. Because of the wide variability in covered benefits, the employee's limited choices may not meet his or her health care needs. It is estimated that 40–70 million Americans have "Swiss cheese policies."[23] These policies have substantial holes or exclusion clauses. Exclusion clauses vary from not covering existing illnesses or high risks—which range from mental illness to pregnancy to diabetes—to not covering certain types of care—which ranges from drugs to organ transplantation to preventive care. Increased deductibles, co-payments, and payment caps are other holes, as are hassle factors. Some of the panoply of hassle factors include requiring the doctor and/or patient to obtain preauthorization for care, justifying emergency care, and limiting care to providers who have a contract with the patient's health plan. Certainly, anyone who has heard an emergency department staffer on the phone begging a health plan clerk for permission to treat a critical patient understands the health plan's powerful authority over the utilization of care.

All plans have some form of holes, but some have more holes than others. This means that in choosing a health plan, the employee must have the knowledge to understand the fine print and the red tape. The employee also needs to be somewhat clairvoyant, anticipating the need for routine care or chemotherapy next year. In short, many factors are beyond the patient's control. Who knows with certainty when he might get sick or when she might lose her job or move outside of the plan's network? After developing a chronic condition six months from now, will he wish he'd chosen a more expensive plan, or that he'd stayed put?

The insertion of fiscal agents and their imposed rules has significantly altered the patient-physician relationship. These changes have introduced a knot of fiduciary, moral, and legal dilemmas, particularly on the physician side of the relationship, which is now informed as much by fiduciary factors as by therapeutic factors. In this new arrangement, physicians ideally are expected to disclose fiduciary information in addition to fulfilling their duty to help and protect the patient. Thus physicians are expected to tell their patients that their income will be greater if they care for the patients' complaints themselves instead of referring them to specialists, if they prescribe a cheaper medicine even though its side effects are more uncomfortable, or if they send the patient's blood work to labs they have invested in.

On the other side of the coin, patients are expected to know about their bodies, to know about treatment options, and to know the benefits covered by their health plan. Because most patients still have limited knowledge about their bodies and about treatment options, most patients don't know whether rightful care has been withheld or the most effective care has been delivered. That is to say, patients are not very effective self-advocates but are still passive recipients of care.

Yet being sick is not like buying a new a toaster, even though health care is a purchased commodity. Sickness induces suffering and a loss of integrity and renders most patients emotionally and cognitively vulnerable. Because they are vulnerable, patients will always need an advocate, one who can aid and protect, who imparts knowledge, and who will help them give voice to their experience. One of the hazards in the new doctor-patient relationship still to be resolved is whether the physician can rightly be expected to fulfill this role of helping the patient through the maze of medical decisions, especially when the physician is also expected to be efficient.

Moreover, in this new relationship, physicians are often caught between their own economic welfare and their patients' needs. For instance, it is safe and right to discharge one day early a healthy thirty-five-year-old male with a broken hip who has a wife and an extended family to support him at home. The eighty-one-year-old widow with a fractured hip, however, is an ethical dilemma for the physician. She is medically stable according to the health plan but has no one to help her at home, lives outside the local boundaries of home-delivered meals, and is too frail to get her own groceries. Should the doctor play it safe therapeutically, keeping her in a skilled nursing facility until she is stronger, knowing that the decision will cost him or her and the facility? Or should the doctor uphold his or her fiduciary responsibilities and send the patient home, knowing that she has a good chance of getting weaker and falling, ending up back in the hospital and, then, in a nursing home for the rest of her life?

Legally, too, the physician is trapped between a rock and a hard place: between the new fiduciary responsibilities and an old, legally sanctioned, standard of care. According to the courts, the physician is expected to treat everyone the same, regardless of ability or inability to pay. Yet the physician has fiduciary permission to shop only from the patients' menu of covered benefits, which vary from health plan to health plan. While courts of law have determined that the physician owes all patients the same degree of skill and care, without regard to others' costs, Morreim concludes that this stance is no longer morally or legally tenable for the physician.[24] He can neither morally nor legally owe what others own and control. To resolve the dilemma, Morreim proposes that the standard of care be divided into two elements. One element, the Standard of Medical Expertise, is the level of knowledge, skill, and diligence the physician owes each patient. Involving his or her professional knowledge, skills, and efforts, this element is fully under the physician's control. The other element, Standard Resource Use, denotes the covered benefits, which entitle the patient to the resources he has paid for.

Although Morreim recommends that these standards be established jointly by physicians, payers, patients, and society at large, she is not advocating a predetermined level of care for all Americans. The solution is a Band-Aid, at best, because it doesn't redress the overarching issues of rising costs and decreasing access to care. At worst, Morreim's solution fosters health care's slide toward tiers of care: upscale care for the wealthy, standard care for those with health insurance, and basic care for people on government assistance. At the bottom are people who have no coverage from any source.

WHO IS RESPONSIBLE FOR CARING FOR THOSE WHO CAN'T PAY?

In the 1950s, when private health insurance had just become established as a customary employee benefit, health care represented about 4 percent of the gross national product (GNP). At that time, most insurance companies used community ratings to price the cost of health insurance, and providers were paid on a cost-plus basis. Then too, physician charges were less regulated. Typically, the wealthy paid more, the less wealthy paid less, and charity was given to those who couldn't pay.

Simply speaking, community rating and cost-plus reimbursement are mechanisms that once helped distribute health care to those who couldn't pay, because they spread the cost of care. Community rating spreads financial risk over a whole community. For instance, white-collar workers and other low-risk groups subsidize high-risk groups such as hard-rock miners and women of childbearing age. In contrast, cost-plus reimbursement enables providers to shift the costs of caring for the uninsured to those with insurance. Cost shifting means that hospitals and physicians incorporate the costs of caring for the uninsured into their fee structure. In other words, cost shifting tacitly makes the insured—more precisely, government and business, the primary purchasers of insurance—responsible for subsidizing the care of the uninsured.

By 2000, no one was happy with health care financing. Community ratings were essentially historical artifacts; managed care made cost shifting generally difficult but failed to control health care costs; and employer coverage was in a state of decline. An estimated 43 million American, 17 percent of noninstitutionalized civilians, were without some form of health insurance, and roughly another 30 million were underinsured. Ironically, about 85 percent of the uninsured population are employed or are dependents of employed persons.[25] Typically, the uninsured are families who earn less than $35,000 annually; early retirees; and people who work for small businesses, in the service industry, or who are self-employed.

A painful paradox is that the uninsured wage earner subsidizes the insured wage earner. Every time he or she buys a car or other items the insured wage earner produces, the uninsured wage earner helps subsidize the coverage of the insured wage earner. Because health benefits are not taxed as income—for example, an employer-paid health benefit worth $500 a month is actually $6,000 in income that's not taxed—the uninsured employee loses twice.

Corporate medicine and managed care have halted providers' ability to redistribute the cost of care. Consequently, care for the uninsured continues to shift to the remaining, overburdened public health clinics; to physician offices that do not depend on managed care contracts; to emergency departments of hospitals; and to out-patient clinics of religious and public agencies. Unfortunately, public funds shrink in the spread of privatization, which is privatization's dark underside. As an anodyne, there is also a growing network of back-room offices staffed by unlicensed practitioners and used mostly by the migrant poor. In the name of good medicine, some states are responding to this by cracking down on back-room offices, passing laws to increase the penalties for practicing without a license, and forming local task forces halt the dispensing of pharmaceuticals.

The bottom line is, it's difficult to get care if one doesn't have health insurance. Despite the uninsured's dependence on public and church-sponsored agencies for care, these services are gravely overburdened. The painful reality is that the uninsured are far less likely than the insured to receive needed preventative care, chronic-disease management, or even treatment for serious medical conditions.

Although public and church-sponsored services are available, they are not easily accessed. The poor face a gauntlet of transportation problems, complicated and difficult qualifying criteria, long waiting lines, and overworked providers. Any one of these barriers to care is overwhelming to someone who doesn't feel well. Moreover, there is little evidence of continuity of care or of a therapeutic relationship. Patients merely see the resident, the intern, or the nurse practitioner scheduled for that shift, and seriously ill patients the doctor would once have hospitalized are now discharged to home or the streets. It's no wonder that patients and providers alike find such care highly alienating and stressful.

The man-as-machine concepts that organize our health care system create significant problems for everyone, but especially for those who don't have health insurance. We cannot blame managed care for this state of affairs. As a society that perceives independent parts, we simply have no mechanism to cover the whole. Accordingly, those who hold the knowledge power have made health an individual commodity and use experience ratings to fracture and segment the market. In the name of efficiency, health insurance is pegged to a constellation of factors—including age, health status, geographic location, and size of employer. We have many well-oiled mechanisms that exclude people from care, even though economic efficiency comes at the price of fairness, trust, and social cohesion.

WHO *IS* RESPONSIBLE FOR PAYING?

Health insurance is the key to accessing health care. Unlike Canadians and Europeans, who have long been protected by some form of universal health insurance, Americans are poorly protected. Health insurance is voluntary for Americans, yet Americans are involuntarily without coverage.

According to the Kaiser Family Foundation,[26] the 1999–2000 population distribution of health insurance was 59 percent employer provided, 5 percent individual, 10 percent Medicaid, and 12 percent Medicare. Fourteen percent of the population was uninsured. Although the majority of Americans receive health insurance through their employment, insurance is voluntary for employers and their employees. This means that coverage is far from guaranteed. People can lose insurance by changes in their employment, marital status, address, and health status. Coverage is also lost if the insurer goes out of business, the employer denies coverage, or workers can no longer afford their portion of the premium costs.

That the bulk of Americans are insured through employer-sponsored health insurance drives a wedge between those with insurance and those without and fosters the sentiment that those without insurance are nonproductive, which is to say, not worthy of coverage. However, the reality is more complicated. The long-term trend has been a decline in employer-sponsored health insurance. Since the late 1970s, health care costs have steadily outpaced the rise in real income, undermining the affordability of health care and increasing the number of uninsured by roughly a million persons per year.[27] The media's focus on rising premium costs to business encourages the pervasive misperception that employers pay most of U.S. health care's costs. Ironically, John Q. Public—not business—pays the bulk of the costs, as shown in figure 6.1.

The business contribution of 34 percent toward total health care costs is about half the amount the public pays. The public pays 60 percent of

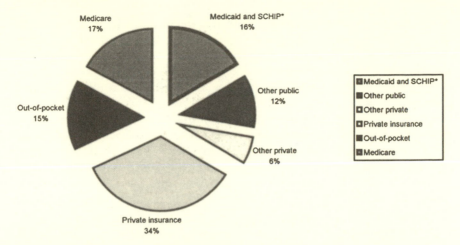

Figure 6.1 The Nation's Health Dollar, 2000
* *State Children's Health Insurance Program*
Source: National Health Care Expenditures. (2000). Pie Charts Depicting the Nation's Health Dollar: 2000—Where It Came From/Where It Went. Available: http://cms.hhs.gov/statistics/nhe/historical/chart.asp

health care costs, through co-pays, deductibles, and other out-of-pocket expenses; through taxes; and through their share of the premium's cost. Actually, the public's cost is probably more. Real pay has stagnated for insured employees since the 1970s, in part to offset soaring insurance premium costs. The uninsured also pay for the health care costs of insured employees, for these costs add to the sticker prices of the toasters, cars, and other goods everyone buys.

THE SYSTEM IS UNFAIR

Everyone pays for health care, but not everyone is included. In Flood's terms, the system is unfair. The structural barriers to obtaining and keeping health insurance; the popular myth that most of the uninsured are unemployed; and the pretension inherent in our employment-based health insurance that premium costs are pegged to utilization are mechanisms that exclude human beings from the care they need. The politically weak and the economically disenfranchised are the most readily excluded, having neither the political clout of special interest groups nor the negotiating power of large business coalitions to leverage their inclusion.

As long as the responsibilities for the delivery and financing of health care are independent functions, what is fair, efficient, or best for the nation's health is irrelevant. Dysfunctional responsibilities foster the game of blame and counterblame. Inherently weakening interpersonal relationships, dysfunctional responsibilities are like fault lines running through the health care system.

Physicians, whose authority stems from their scientific knowledge, are responsible for balancing a patient's medical needs with the payers' financial requirements. However, CEOs of businesses and insurance companies operate within an entirely different context, whose value—economic growth—is often at odds with the value of health. Accountable to their stockholders, the CEOs' responsibilities are fiduciary, and it is outside health care's conceptual framework to ask, How can medical and fiduciary responsibilities be balanced? Meanwhile, fertility and end-of-life issues, genetic engineering, the growing number of uninsured, and emerging concerns regarding population health issues increasingly are matters of public concern. Like the blind men and the elephant, each one advocating his position, no one is responsible for the health of the whole.

Unfortunately, it is our habit to understand things by taking them apart, to isolate in order to control. Health care's unfairness is not an accident but emerges from the devolution of modernity's separation of self from other. That stakeholders are perceived as independent rather than interdependent provokes competition rather than collaboration, reinforces privilege and authority for stakeholders who claim expert knowledge, and leads to inadequate access and poor quality of care for those with less power. The organization of health care compels each special interest group to protect its own interests. Organized to separate, reduce, and exclude, the modern organization of the health care system ineluctably fosters special interest groups and reinforces economic gamesmanship and piecemeal legislation.

To use Wilber's language, we can't integrate I, We, and It. Modernity's self-centered, reductionistic, either/or perspective makes it impossible to generate a health care system that is fair. Objectifying each other, I lose sight of We. Fragmented, we reduce our choices to opposing actions and lose our balance. When the whole is eclipsed by its parts, one of us loses: Either I care for my neighbors and disregard my own needs, or I obligate my neighbors to care for me and I disregard their needs. In actuality, both of us eventually lose.

THE WOUNDED SYSTEM

There will always be a healer-patient relationship. However, recent advances in biotechnology; new knowledge regarding behavioral, social, and environmental determinants of health; and managed care have made many of the elements in Parsons's sick role obsolete and have forced the

traditional doctor-patient relationship into a state of flux. The destructur-
ing of the traditional doctor-patient relationship, once the keystone of
health care, has exposed serious contradictions and disconnections in the
less-apparent whole.

Just as an overdose of medication makes a person sicker, incessant economic growth and an overdependence on technology have wounded
health care. Reducing care to objective biochemical events and profit-
maximizing technological interventions disconnects the subject from the
object, the patient from the healer, the self from others, and morals from
measures.

Health care's contradictions and disconnections are not surprising
because they originate within health care's theoretical framework—the
modern worldview—and are replicated and amplified by the self and the
market economy, two of the other systems in the nested hierarchy. Health
means wholeness. But health care's theoretical foundation—reductionism, materialism, and self-centeredness—contradicts the meaning of
health. Due to this fragmented way of thinking, health care is wounded.
Physicians are responsible for producing health, but the best they can do
is treat one patient at a time. Moreover, managed care organizations
strictly limit their responsibility to their covered populations. It is outside
modernity's conceptual framework for either stakeholder to ask, Who is
responsible for the care of the whole?

When the nested hierarchy is viewed through the lens of economics,
another set of disconnections and contradictions is exposed. Within the
context of health care, managed care has made physicians responsible for
balancing the patient's medical needs with the payers' financial requirements. However, CEOs of businesses and insurance companies, the purchasers and payers, operate within an entirely different context, whose
value—economic growth—is often at odds with the value of health.
Accountable to their boards of directors and stockholders, the CEOs'
responsibilities are fiduciary. Because the balance sheet specifies the right
decision, their decisions become the cliché, It's nothing personal, it's just
business.

WHO *IS* RESPONSIBLE?

To a very large extent, systems shape behavior. People inside health
care—doctors, patients, insurance administrators, and so forth—don't
function as independent agents but behave in accordance with their roles,
and these roles are defined in accordance with broader cultural variables
that emanate from the prevailing worldview. Completing the circle, a
worldview is the product of human thought.

When we forget that social systems are the product of human thought,
we become, as Peter Senge says, prisoners of the system. It's circular: dys-

functional systems ↔ dysfunctional roles ↔ dysfunctional thought. To show that we are the victim and not the culprit when something goes wrong, we need something to blame. Senge refers to this prisoner/blame habit as a "learning disability."[28] That is, we don't learn from our mistakes but instead keep doing the very things that create the dysfunction.

CHANGING THE SYSTEM

The escape is to *see* both the constraints imposed by the system and the thought that spawns our actions. The challenge, however, is to rewire health care, to integrate what thought has fractured into a coherent whole. Ineluctably, we do depend upon one another. Systemic change is based on a paradoxical awareness: that our own well-being depends upon the well-being of others. Relationships connect people to people and systems to systems. Neither the doctor, the patient, nor the payer is independent of the other two.

Responsibilities affect the integrity of the relationships. *Responsibility* means the ability to answer, and being responsible means having the authority, the resources, and the knowledge to act, or to respond. In contrast, accountability means claiming ownership for the consequences of one's responses. When the constraints imposed by the system result in dysfunctional relationships, or when individuals don't claim ownership for the consequences of their actions, integrity is compromised.

As a society, we can no longer afford to ignore the dysfunctional responsibilities and health care's inherent unfairness. Americans are leery of health care reform, however. The subject is highly contentious and, so far, fraught with failure. Trust and trustworthiness are eclipsed when competition is the name of the game. Firmly believing that any improvement will be costly, the public is afraid of losing what it already has. The proposed incremental reforms of employment-based health insurance, vouchers, and modifications to Medicare and Medicaid are merely yesterday's thinking. Incremental reform can't make health care fairer or guarantee coverage for all of us. Instead, incremental reform simply adds to the present crazy quilt of conflicting and incoherent policies and guarantees more of the same: more losers in health care's game of economic musical chairs.

In systems language, incremental reform of health insurance is merely tampering with the processes inside of health care. Incremental insurance reform can't make health care more efficient or effective or halt health care's vicious economic cycles and soaring costs. Because insurance reform doesn't add critical balancing loops, it can't check the financial incentives built into the health care system that reinforce economic growth.

CHANGING OUR RELATIONSHIPS

If we are to make the health care system fair, we need to change our thinking. Fair means the entire population is guaranteed access to a pre-determined level of care across a continuum of health conditions. We can't solve today's fairness problems using the same concepts that reinforce health care's contradictory values and severed relationships. The challenge of health care reform is not to create another round of winners and losers, or to persuade the public to give up beneficial care, but to integrate what modernity has differentiated; what Wilber refers to as I, We, and It. This is shorthand for self, others, and things; for me, morals, and money.

Integration means new responsibilities. Stakeholders can't respond in old ways; the answers from their memory-version of reality are worn out and dysfunctional. New responsibilities mean new knowledge, new authority, and access to new resources. This is tricky because health care is one system in a nested hierarchy: self, health care, market economy, and worldview. In other words, there are levels of integration, just as our five senses, our muscles, and our nerves cooperate to keep us balanced and upright. Integration means not only a new balance of traditional clinical and fiduciary responsibilities but new, health-producing responsibilities for corporate and government leaders. Even though very few Americans can authorize policy and spending changes, each one of us is responsible for what we think is fair. Each one of us is responsible for what we think about, the way we care for, and what we wish for people who are different from ourselves.

CHANGING OUR THINKING

We can't afford the high costs of victim blaming because we can't escape the consequences of our relationships. Inexorably, we are connected to one another and to the things we make. The challenge is to see the whole and to connect political, institutional, and personal responsibilities in such a way that what is right and good for the individual is also right and good for the whole.

S. I. Hayakawa speaks to perceiving the world in a more holistic way in an essay titled "The Revision of Vision":

Vision shares with speech the distinction of being the most important of the means by which we apprehend reality. To cease looking at things atomistically in visual experience and to see relatedness means, among other things, to lose in our social experience, as Mr. Kepes argues, the deluded self-importance of absolute "individualism" in favor of social relatedness and interdependence. When we structuralize the primary impacts of experience differently, we shall structuralize the world differently.[29]

QUESTIONS FOR THE READER

1. When your condition can't be cured, who is responsible for caring for you? What kind of care do you want?

2. When you can no longer take care of yourself, who do you expect to care for you—your children, your spouse, church members, the government?

3. Who do you expect to pay for this care—yourself, your children, your health insurance, the government?

4. If your care requires lots of expensive resources that you can't readily afford, which of today's hard choices will you pick: institutionalizing a sick child or divorcing a sick spouse in order to receive Medicaid, or draining the family physically, financially, and emotionally?

5. If your affliction is chronic, what resources would you find beneficial? What is your responsibility toward managing this condition?

6. What kind of a physician do you want? One who is aggressive and high tech; one who includes you in the decision-making process; one who has empathy and respect for your age, socioeconomic status, and so forth; or something else?

7. If you live or work in a toxic, high-stress environment, drive an unsafe car, or use hazardous products, who is responsible when you become sick or are injured?

8. Who is responsible for providing health care and paying for this care if you (or others) make bad choices or have bad luck?

9. To what extent are you responsible for the well-being of others?

10. To what extent do your neighbors have an obligation to provide the assistance needed to meet our collective needs? To what extent does society have an obligation to meet your needs?

11. How do we become responsible for our lives—for what we say and do, for how we think and feel—knowing that there are limits to what others can do for us, yet knowing that we need one another?

CHAPTER 7

A Call to Be Whole

No product can be better than the system that produces it.
No system can be better than the relationships among its stakeholders.
And all relationships hang by the thin thread of conversation.
                                                              —Barbara Sowada

THE PRECARIOUS SYSTEM

The multiple, conflicting, inconsistent answers to What is health? What is care? How much is enough? and Who is responsible? tell us that the health care system is in trouble. So do the rising costs of health care, the inequities of access, the inadequacies of technology to care for those with chronic and life-threatening conditions, and the inability of biomedicine to care for the health of the population. These are all signs of systemic instability.

Unstable systems are dysfunctional, and dysfunctional systems are unproductive. Systemic instability means that the system is not accomplishing its purpose, necessary elements are not included, or the relationships among its elements are not cooperative and resources are wasted. All three causes of instability are perturbing the current health care system.

Our earlier inquiries illuminated the concepts, the stakeholders, and the elements—healer, patient, remedy, and cause—that compose the health care system. So where do we direct our efforts for health care reform, and why do we choose certain interventions over others? To clearly see the cause and effect of our efforts requires that we return to our Russian doll analogy—in which each doll in a nested set is enveloped by a larger doll (Figure 2.1)—and unpack the nested hierarchy of systems: self, health care, market economy, and worldview.

PRINCIPLES OF SYSTEMIC CHANGE

Systems are defined by the organization of their elements. The arrangement of the elements forms and informs the structure and function of the system. As the Russian doll analogy depicts, systems are not independent entities but are parts in larger wholes. Each system depends upon the inputs of other systems, and each needs other systems to receive its outputs. Directly or indirectly affecting one another, each system behaves the way it does because of the actions of the others. Each system needs the others to be itself.

In our dynamic universe, there is a constant flow of information, material, and energy. In short, things change. Perturbations happen. Depending upon the nature of the perturbation, systems can take one of four paths: preservation, adaptation, dissolution, and evolution (transcendence). In a dynamic universe, all systems are poised between absolute regularity and absolute chaos.

Like the elasticity of a rubber band, *preservation* allows individual systems to be perturbed yet return to the status quo. Systems are designed to tolerate a certain amount of variation. For example, a finely tuned system like the heart can slow down to as few as 40 beats per minute or speed up to around 200 beats per minute, depending upon the body's needs, without any damage. The propensity to return to equilibrium is what lets us recover from disease and injury. The more complex the system, or the more feedback loops it contains, the more disorder the system can tolerate. This is because the more feedback loops it has, the more ways it has to respond to perturbations.

Adaptation, on the other hand, implies a kind of plasticity, a remodeling of the system while conserving its defining structure and function. Obesity and a child's growing to adulthood are two examples of adaptation. Adaptation means that the system can maintain its integrity yet fit within a larger whole. Adaptation is a survival feature. Like preservation, adaptation is a function of the system's structure, for it is the ability to adjust internal mechanisms that let a system survive a changing outer world.

With strong perturbations, however, the result is quite different. Perturbations strong enough to overcome the system's equilibrium dislodge the system from its energy trough, causing the system to dissolve or evolve.

Chemists depict stable compounds as resting in an energy trough. Once dislodged from the energy trough, the compound follows the path of least resistance until equilibrium, or stability, is restored. To dislodge a compound is to destroy the original pattern so the compound either dissolves into its more basic parts or evolves into a more complex entity. For example, aerobic exercise tips fat molecules out of their energy trough and reduces them to the basic components CO_2 and H_2O. In contrast, when fat molecules are tipped out of their energy trough in the presence of estrogen, the short-chain fatty acids are reassembled into the more complex entity cholesterol.

Dissolution occurs when the perturbation exceeds the system's equilibrium. As all systems seek equilibrium, dissolution means that equilibrium has been found at a lower energy level. In other words, the new system is a less complex whole; for example, CO_2 is a simpler molecule than a fat molecule.

However, if the causes and conditions are favorable, the perturbation may evoke *evolution*. Evolution, which is the reverse of dissolution, means the synthesis of a novel and more complex system. What were once autonomous parts have re-formed into a more complex whole, as fatty acids $\rightarrow$ cholesterol. The new system is more than the sum of its parts. The new system is richer in information and energy than its predecessors, with its own pattern and capacity for preservation and adaptation.

THE PRECARIOUS HEALTH CARE SYSTEM

Just as some types of inborn errors of metabolism take years to cause physical symptoms, health care has only recently begun to experience pathological symptoms arising from modernity's dominant concepts: reductionism, materialism, determinism, and self-centeredness. Like chickens and eggs, health care and these concepts keep emerging from and producing each other, again and again.

The concepts themselves are not inherently flawed. They gave birth to the scientific revolution and developed the benefits of modern medicine. The problem is that the stakeholders with the knowledge power assiduously restrict health care and health care reform to reductionism, materialism, and self-centeredness.

Overplayed, these concepts have become liabilities, and the result is ever-more-specialized and fragmented care, an overdependence on biotechnology, a blind eye toward the social and environmental determinants of health, and piecemeal efforts at health care reform. Overplayed, these concepts amplify selfish individualism and economic competition at the expense of social relatedness and interdependence. Overplayed, these concepts are serious perturbations, bringing health care to a tipping point, a precarious place where systemic stability is easily and irretrievably lost.

We all feel these perturbations: debilitating health care costs and deteriorating quality and access; a widening of the schisms between public and private medicine and between mind, body, and spirit; intense, cutthroat competition among the stakeholders; and fears of being excluded or dying alone, in pain, and broke.

THE ILLUSION OF CONTROL

National polls such as the one conducted by NPR/Kaiser/Kennedy School[1] show that Americans favor building on the current system. Adaptation, or piecemeal reform, seems safe. Remembering President Clinton's comprehensive health plan and its massive failure, the public is rightfully leery. Doing something small and contained, such as subsidizing drug costs for the elderly or making it easier or harder for patients to sue their HMOs, doesn't raise taxes and, as the ad said, "keeps the government out of our medicine chest." In short, piecemeal reform offers the illusion of control.

When we look at modernity's most distinguishing concept—the part is more important than the whole—adaptation seems reasonable. From modernity's perspective, fixing the broken part and attending to the concern of the day are logical behaviors. Looking a little deeper, however, we see that when the parts are more important than the whole, the whole is poorly integrated; and patients, providers, payers, and purchasers are functioning relatively independently.

Just as each blind man described his part as the true elephant, the stakeholders are separated by different ideas regarding the meaning of health and the purpose of health care, different goals, and different understandings of biomedicine's capacity. Moreover, because there are at least five definitions of health in play, the purpose of health care is indefinite and fungible, allowing powerful stakeholders to play on the public's fears and mold the purpose of health care to suit their particular desires. Unable to see the whole, each part tries to protect itself by controlling the others.

ADAPTATION'S FALSE PROMISES

The illusion of safety comes at a cost. Managed care exemplifies the cost and the failure of incremental reform. Essentially, managed care was an attempt to improve cooperation among payers, purchasers, and providers. Beginning in the early 1970s, business was no longer willing to absorb health care costs into its production costs. Distressed that health care had rebuffed its earlier efforts at cooperative control, business played its hand. By the time Bill Clinton became president, the courts and the legislatures had dismantled many of the laws and regulations that providers had accumulated to dominate the health care market place. By 1994, health care reform had defaulted to managed care, signified by risk-sharing methods of reimbursement, more oversight and rules, and additional layers of bureaucracy for tighter control. Economic and political power had largely shifted from providers to payers and purchasers, and health care had assumed all the characteristics of a large corporation, with a profit margin among the highest of any industry (see Table 7.1).

Table 7.1
Axes of Change in the U.S. Health Care System

Dimensions	From Provider-Driven	To Buyer-Driven
Ideological	Sacred trust in doctors	Distrust of doctors values, decisions, competence
Economic	Carte blanche to do what seems best; power to set fees; incentives to specialize, to develop techniques Informal array of cross-subsidizations for teaching, research, charity care, community services	Fixed prepayment or contract, with accountability for decisions and their efficacy Elimination of cost-shifting, payment only for services contracted.
Political	Extensive legal and administrative power to define and carry out professional work without competition and to shape the organization and economics of medicine	Minimal legal and administrative power to do professional work but no power to shape the organization and economics of services
Clinical	Exclusive control of clinical decision-making Emphasis on state-of-the-art specialized interventions; lack of interest in prevention, primary care, and chronic care	Close monitoring of clinical decisions, their cost, and efficacy. Emphasis on prevention, primary care, and functioning; minimization of high-tech and specialized interventions
Technical	Political and economic incentives to develop new technologies in protected markets	Political and economic disincentives to develop new technologies

Source: Light, D. W. (1991, Fall). Professionalism as a countervailing power. *Journal of Health Politics, Policy and Law,* 16(3), 499–506.

CANCEROUS ECONOMIC GROWTH

The shift from a provider-driven to a buyer-driven system did not control health care costs. It couldn't. On one hand, like all other businesses, health care expects its profits to grow. On the other hand, efficiency measures inside health care can't halt rising health care costs. Total costs depend upon the amount of resources flowing into the system, and the U.S. system does not have a shutoff valve. That requires a global budget, and the shift from provider-driven to buyer-driven system didn't supply the missing shutoff valve (a balancing loop, in systems language).

The shift from provider-driven to buyer-driven was the adaptation imposed on the health care system. To be consistent with the systemic changes, stakeholders adapted as well, by adjusting the flow of resources among themselves, further intensifying the competition instead of improving cooperation.

The problem with adaptive economic solutions is that health care has an overabundance of unchecked reinforcing loops. In any system with too many unchecked reinforcing loops, small actions escalate into ever-larger consequences. In the absence of a global budget, tampering with processes inside of health care amplifies the effects of reinforcing loops. Because reinforcing feedback loops have a snowballing effect, the shift made costs, quality, and access problems worse rather than better.

Without a global budget, or a balancing loop between health care and the market economy, economic adaptations can only backfire. Cost containment efforts can only bring more of the same: heightened competition, cutbacks in services deemed unprofitable, and greater risk segregation. Those people typically most in need of health care's services are the most likely to be excluded. After all, in this modern, self-centered game, health care is a commodity for personal use. Why should the well, the young, and the rich pay for the care of the sick, the elderly, and the poor—or so they ask?

The stark reality is, however, that unchecked growth eventually destabilizes all systems. Just as a cancer can only grow so large before it kills its host, limits are eventually encountered. Once past the tipping point, the health care system will fall apart. Although it is counterintuitive, health care costs can't be redressed with financial solutions alone. By themselves, financial solutions will further destabilize the existing system.

UNPACKING THE NESTED HIERARCHY OF SYSTEMS

To understand why adaptive solutions for health care are destined to fail we need to unpack health care as one system inside a nested hierarchy of systems: the self, health care, the market economy, and an organizing worldview.

Systems incorporate their organizing worldview and are internally consistent with the organizing worldview. Internally consistent is depicted by the Russian doll analogy and means that the behavior of the market economy and health care is compatible with and can be explained by the worldview's exemplars. Even the way we apprehend our reality is in accordance with the organizing worldview, for we, too, are included in this nested hierarchy.

Because nested systems are internally consistent, we should see the same issues replicated in both health care and our market economy, and we do. Modern concepts reinforce our habit of taking things apart to understand them, of isolating in order to control, of objectifying in order to count, of valuing growth at any cost. Matter is all that matters. Material wealth is the product of the market economy, and material health is the product of the health care system.

Unfortunately, because matter is all that matters, the social and environmental costs, such as latchkey kids, rising joblessness, and global warming, are automatically excluded from the market system's actual production costs. All that counts in our economic system is the overall production of goods and services, transacted in monetary terms. Likewise, a material view of the world causes health care to function as a biological repair shop. Because modernity excludes the nonbiological determinants of health, the environmental, social, behavioral, and spiritual determinants of health important to the health needs of the whole population and those with chronic and life-threatening diseases are automatically excluded from the production line.

Adaptation means that a system maintains its integrity yet continues to fit within a larger whole. In other words, adaptation preserves health care's defining structure and function, first by holding us to our modern understanding of healer, patient, remedy, and cause, and second by holding us to the market production model. To fit within the constraints imposed by the modern worldview, adaptation means finding new technological ways to fix and prevent biological flaws in individual persons. It also means, as managed care demonstrates, that health care is measured out, packaged as a consumer good, and paid for in units of service.

Adaptation is not reform. Adaptation can only amplify what is overplayed, for adaptation doesn't let us escape modernity's dominant concepts: reductionism, materialism, determinism, and self-centeredness. The problem is that unless we escape modernity's dominant concepts, we can't effectively or efficiently redress population health issues, humanely care for those with life-threatening and chronic diseases, or control health care costs.

SEEING MODERNITY'S TRAP

Systems, as we've said, are organized to preserve themselves. Having incorporated a worldview, a system uses that worldview to protect itself, for the worldview is self-sealing. That is, the system uses its worldview to validate the information it recognizes and uses the information to prove the validity of the worldview. In short, systems protect themselves by recognizing some information but not all information. If the information is not consistent with the worldview, the information won't be allowed in or even recognized.

Because modernity conditions us to see parts, not wholes, we see health care as an independent system. We do not see health care as one system in a nested hierarchy of systems: self, health care, market economy, and worldview. We can't. When we are conditioned to see independent systems, our apprehension of reality ricochets between two extremes. One is that everything is independent and stands alone. It's the cliché, we can't see the forest for the trees. Overwhelmed by trees, we lose sight of the forest. At the other extreme, everything is collapsed into one entity. Overwhelmed by the forest, we can't distinguish the individual trees. Either way, we perceive things as independent entities.

When things are perceived as independent entities, connections drop out of sight. Simply put, relationships and interdependence among the nested systems don't exist according to modern exemplars. For example, modernity blinds us to the connection between health care and the market economy. As a result, we can neither see that these two systems are connected by an information loop that reinforces economic growth and the commodification of health, nor see that the balancing loop, necessary for systemic stability, is missing.

The trap is that even when the exemplars no longer work, the self-sealing nature of the worldview continues to protect itself. In short, human beings become prisoners of the system. For example, by virtue of our role inclusion, health care influences our beliefs, determines our experiences, and validates our behavior regarding health. However, as modernity inherently protects itself, any information about health care that is not compatible with modern exemplars is simply not recognized or is discounted. Paradoxically, the rejection is always personal. People advocating relationships, interdependence, or information that is not compatible with modern exemplars are disregarded or find themselves subtly and explicitly excluded by those holding the knowledge power.

UNHEALTHY BOUNDARIES

In everyday language, when people take in information that is disrespectful or harmful or when they manipulate information in order to control others, they are thought of as having boundary issues. There is a remarkable similarity between unhealthy systems and unhealthy personal relationships. Both have boundary issues. It is impossible to have a healthy personal relationship with someone whose boundaries are too rigid or too porous. Overly rigid boundaries close people off to new information. We refer to such people as controlling, rigid, or well-defended. Boundaries that are too porous, however, let all information in equally, leaving people feeling engulfed and controlled by others. People with overly porous boundaries are often labeled codependent.

Like the saying "good fences make good neighbors," healthy boundaries provide enough protection so people feel safe being real with one another. Paradoxically, when people feel safe in their vulnerability, information that threatens the status quo can be let in. People don't need to wall themselves off from new information by blaming others, controlling others, or simply withdrawing. In this paradoxical space, love and respect thrive.

That said, unhealthy boundaries breed distrust, confusion, and self-centeredness. People can't afford to be real with one another. When information is limited, there is a lot of game playing, rumor, and gossip as people try to figure out what is going on. The welfare of the whole is ignored, for a distrustful environment conditions people to look out for number one, and everything that happens is perceived as an attack against or a validation of the self. There is a preoccupation with control; and to protect themselves, people spend an inordinate amount of time blaming or trying to control others, or they withdraw to a professional stance.

Ironically, this behavior reinforces health care's guiding principle: The part is more important than the whole. It is a vicious cycle. The system has assumed a life of its own because the people animating it are closed to new information vital to understanding their codependent condition. Without new information—and when boundaries are unhealthy, the system is averse to new information—the options for new understandings and new ways of behaving remain closed. The dilemma is painful: To escape the threatening turmoil of the status quo means new information; however, new information is automatically discounted as being threatening.

THE POWER OF STRUCTURE

The deeper purpose of unpacking the nested hierarchy is to illuminate the power inherent in a system's structure. Human-made systems are very much like organic molecules. For example, health care is divided into separate specialties and organized by product lines. Managers pay a lot of attention to the structure of tasks that people perform. The division of labor and the organization of work are like the arrangement of atoms in chemical molecules. As the energy bonds hold chemical molecules together, human beings are held together through our roles. These roles, informed by the incorporated worldview, tightly govern our behavior. There is a reason people often say a system has a life of its own. It takes a lot of energy to dislodge a human-made system from its energy trough.

WE KNOW WHAT IS NEEDED TO MAKE HEALTH CARE MORE WHOLE

Having unpacked the nested hierarchy and seen the ways the health care system preserves itself and protects its organizing worldview, we can more deeply appreciate the power inherent in a system's structure. It is the deeply embedded power of thought that makes transformative change so difficult.

The poignant reality is that we do know what is needed to make health care more whole. In systems language, the solution lies in establishing new boundaries and incorporating new feedback loops into the structure of health care. New feedback loops are more than economic off switches; they are mechanisms that change relationships by redistributing economic resources; by incorporating the nonmaterial (spiritual, social, and behavioral) determents of health; and by reforming responsibilities. The purpose of these systemic alterations is to contain health care costs and to improve access and quality, or, as Flood would say, to make the health care system more effective, efficient, and fair.

In systems language, we know the three high-leverage points. One is the insertion of a balancing feedback loop—a global budget—between health care and the market economy. This controls costs without damaging access and quality. The second is to distinguish population health from individual medical care. While this redraws health care's boundaries, it also clarifies its purpose. The third leverage point involves the distinction of prevention and acute, chronic, and life-threatening needs so that the right mix of medical, social, and behavioral resources is delivered. These levers have already been invented, but they aren't widely publicized.

A Global Budget

Global budget concepts are the framework for the Josephine Butler United States Health Service Act (H.R. 1374),[2] introduced by Congressman Ronald Dellums and his associates in 1977. The purpose of this act was to transcend the liabilities of the current system by establishing a United States health service. A major redesign of health care, the act makes health care a public service. To provide high-quality comprehensive health care for all Americans, the Dellums bill calls for predetermined levels of diagnostic, therapeutic, preventive, rehabilitative, environmental, and occupational health services; ambulance, homemaking, behavioral, and social services; drugs; and dental and vision care.

The services are financed through capitation and progressive taxation of individuals and corporations, limiting the profits of providers, purveyors, and payers. Access is universal; all geographic areas are assured of adequate service, including those now underserved; and continuity of care is assured by linking local facilities to regional special-care facilities. Publicly elected regional and national boards are responsible for the planning and governance of the Health Service.

Improving the Care of Chronic and Life-Threatening Sickness

To improve the care of chronic and life-threatening diseases, the Institute of Medicine's 2001 report *Crossing the Quality Chasm: A New Health System for the Twenty-first Century*[3] also recommends significant systemic changes to the health care system. Understanding that quality is a systems property, the institute proposes a more holistic approach to the traditional doctor-patient relationship. Briefly, the proposed systemic changes include customizing care to fit patients' and families' social, behavioral, and financial needs; development of "best practice" strategies and standardized treatment protocols to reduce the present misuse, underuse, and overuse of resources; and the development and strengthening of multidiscipline teams that include a doctor, a nurse, a social worker, and other therapists. Because about 40 percent of patients are afflicted with more than one chronic condition, the plan also calls for integrating information systems in order to coordinate the care delivered across multiple treatment settings. The plan also proposes a realignment of financial incentives so that physicians are paid for the time-consuming coordination and management of care.

MediCaring

MediCaring, a demonstration project of the Center to Improve the Care of the Dying, presents a holistic approach to caring for patients with life-threatening diseases.[4] Life-threatening means that patients are nearing the end of life, the final two to three years. Briefly, MediCaring calls for an interdisciplinary approach, integration of diverse services, patient and family counseling and support, symptom control and functional maintenance, and continuity and coordination of care that is tailored to meet the individual patient's needs. In short, care is designed to help the patient live in dignity and comfort until the end.

MediCaring's designers, too, recognize that quality is a systems property. Their proposed goals are systemic changes. One of the goals is to reshape Medicare's payment policy, whose fee-for-service structure discourages the integrated management of care and encourages acute over palliative treatment. Another is to broaden eligibility requirements, using severity of illness measurements associated with chronic diseases and frailty instead of hospice's restrictive prognosis. The final goal is to change the attitudes and behaviors of providers away from the professional stance to one of mutual respect and reciprocal caring.

Health Canada

Health Canada is an example of a system that addresses population health. Signed into law in 1994, the purpose of Health Canada is to improve the health of the whole population and to reduce inequities in health status among Canadian population groups by attending to the social, environmental, and behavioral determinants of health.[5] Health Canada is a complex, multifaceted program that engages citizens at individual, corporate, provincial, and federal levels and entails new accountabilities across public and private sectors normally not associated with health. It provides national leadership to develop health policy, promote healthy lifestyles and disease prevention, and enforce health regulations. Decisions are evidence-based, and quality is measured in terms of outcomes as opposed to traditional criteria: inputs, processes, procedures, and products. Health Canada is not a quantitative model that can predict either cause or effect with mathematical certainty. Instead, it is a work in progress that focuses on the health of the whole population.

The Canadian health care system is not responsible for all of the determinants of health, so the model redefines health care's boundaries. Although other social institutions contribute to the population's health, health care's role is prominent and significant. Consequently, Health Canada is committed to maintaining Canada's health insurance system, which makes comprehensive services universally available to Canadian citizens.

HUMAN BEINGS AND THEIR SYSTEMS ARE MUTUALLY ENFOLDED

It should now be obvious that we don't need to invent any wheels to reform our health care system. What is best for the nation's health is largely known, as are the general improvements needed to better the U.S. health care system's international ranking: first in costs, and thirty-seventh in keeping people healthy. That we know what is needed but are resistant to health care reform brings us to the tightest knot in our inquiry: the system referred to as the self.

The purpose of unpacking the nested hierarchy of systems is to clearly see that the health care system is not an independent entity, but that human beings and their systems are mutually enfolded. They are mutually enfolded because human thought produces human-made systems, and human-made systems, by virtue of our role inclusion, direct our thoughts and actions, as illustrated in figure 7.1.

A hologram is good analogy for describing human beings and their systems: The worldview we see in one system is replicated in the others. A biological analogy is, each cell in the body—in the liver, blood, bone, and so forth—contains the same genetic pattern. Basically, we can think of the nested hierarchy as one very complex system in which, as in all complex systems, the whole and each part behave in ways that are consistent with one another and with their organizing worldview.

THE INERTIA OF THE STATUS QUO

Because our sense of self as a separate entity is also modern product, it follows that our thoughts and actions are consistent with modern concepts. Our nervous system is hardwired with modern concepts, which is why social scientists describe the self as an independent entity imbued with inalienable rights and motivated by self-interest. Although self-interest refers to maximizing the "good," which in a material world typically

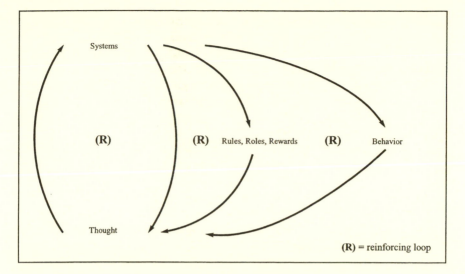

Figure 7.1 Human-Made Systems, Thought, and Behavior Are Mutually
Reinforcing

defaults to material acquisition, the pursuit of self-interest also includes
minimizing the "bad," or keeping it outside the self's boundaries.

As long as these concepts are largely taken for granted by significant
numbers of Americans, we will continue to incorporate modern concepts
into the roles, rules, and rewards that comprise our human-made systems.
Having designed modern concepts into the roles, rules, and rewards that
inform the structures of our systems, our social systems then subtly and
explicitly reinforce behavior that is consistent with modern concepts.

As we've seen, health care is a closed system. Like all closed systems,
health care limits the behaviors a person has in terms of roles; it even limits the thoughts a person can perceive and advocate. Because health care is
part of a nested hierarchy that is also a closed system, novel information
can be repudiated at any level of the hierarchy. At each level, however, all
information is not equally novel. For instance, information that is novel or
threatening to health care may be acceptable to the economic system, or
information that threatens my rights, privileges, and responsibilities as a
doctor may not threaten yours as a managed care executive.

Because novel information needs to pass through layers of barriers and
affects each system differently, it is important to see each system in the
nested hierarchy as an autonomous entity and to not collapse the whole
into the health care system. We have layers of barriers to new information.
Paradoxically, due to our tendencies to collapse everything into health
care and take our worldview for granted, status quo–protecting barriers
are largely ignored or misunderstood. They are perceived as outside of us.

It's time to unpack the layers of methods we use to preserve our view of our selves, that is, to avoid changing our minds.

MINE VERSUS OBJECT

As we've said, when it comes to health care, most Americans are hard-wired with modern concepts. Consequently, we perceive the world as separate parts and ourselves as independent entities. It follows, then, that what isn't "mine" is perceived as an object outside of me, which modernity tells me I can control. This perception of "mine" versus "object" ("I" and "it" in Wilber's terms) is a block to true health care reform. It is our habit to reject novel information and preserve modern concepts by objectifying others and believing we can control any object.

ADAPTIVE CHANGES

Adaptive changes are consistent with "mine" thinking. Adaptive changes seem safe and logical because adaptation does not threaten the status quo. Nonadaptive behavior would be judged false or threatening according to modern concepts, whereas what is known, or mine, seems safe. To protect our worldview, we continue to dream up new reimbursement procedures, new accounting methods, more layers of control and regulation, corporatization, reengineering, customer service programs, quality report cards, and advertising campaigns.

All of these adaptations are consistent with modern concepts, so they feel familiar and safe. We have kept the bad, the unknown, and the foreign outside ourselves. Moreover, when our adaptations fail to control costs or to improve quality and access, as they inevitably do, we can still feel safe. Because our modern, objective worldview has detached us from one another and the things we make, we simply tighten control or blame others, citing poor planning, lack of leadership, or poor cooperation.

OBJECTIVE, OR MECHANISTIC, CHANGES

Objective, or mechanistic, changes are consistent with object thinking. Because modernity conditions us to perceive independent parts, we view health care as an object totally separate from us. We try to re-form health care as if it were made of Tinkertoys. (If health care were an isolated structure built of inert rods and connecting pieces, systemic re-form would be quite easy. To alter boundaries, add new balancing loops, modify resources, and improve relationships would simply entail adding new rods and connecting pieces.) People who perceive health care as an object focus on piecemeal, structural changes. They attempt to fix the broken part and either don't see or attempt to suppress the effect structural changes have on people. Thus, as exemplified by the steady stream of new legislation to fix the problems of managed care, another round of structural changes is imposed to cope with the inevitable fallout.

When what isn't "mine" is perceived as an object outside of me, other people tend to become objects in our minds, too. They become tools, "Its," as Wilber would say, to be used or manipulated or controlled in the pursuit of our self-interest. From this mechanistic perspective, we see others as Its and don't see the reciprocal relationship between structure and behavior. People's behavior is simply another part in the machine, another part that can be fixed in isolation of others' roles and rules.

Health care organizations are rightfully concerned about quality and customer service. They want patients to feel cared for. Consequently, a lot of time and money is spent on customer-service training. Yet having nurses provide tender, loving care is as much a staffing issue as it is an attitude issue. If management attempts to improve quality by sending nurses to customer-service training but doesn't change its lean and mean staffing processes, nurses will continue to feel rushed, overworked, depressed, and cynical toward both patients and management. As roles are built into the system, so are quality and caring. Responding to call lights more quickly and preventing medication errors is more a function of available time than it is of smiling and having the right attitude.

Object, independent-parts thinking turns other people into Its and eclipses the tight relationship between human behavior and a system's processes. The eclipse conceals the fact that to change either the behavior or the process is to change both of them. In actuality, role behavior can't change without structural changes, and structural changes can't avoid altering roles, rules, and rewards; the organization of work; and the networks of interpersonal relationships.

Our dilemma, using Wilber's language, is that we see I and It, but It is perceived as disconnected from us, and We (the intersubjective relationship) is not in sight. The unfortunate net result of our inability to perceive relationships and interdependence is that we don't remember that we are connected to one another and to the things we make. As a result, we attempt to change objects to preserve the illusion of control and the status quo of independent parts.

DISCOUNTING CURRENT REALITY

Current reality is the actual state we are in right now. Current reality is often described as being in the moment—neither mentally replaying the past nor projecting into the future. In current reality, the automatic pilot has been turned off. Briefly, current reality includes but is more than objective data—the things we can see, touch, smell, taste, and hear, and count, measure, and weigh—because it also includes being truthful about our emotions, our beliefs, our reasoning, and our interpretation of the current experience.

This is why stories are as important as numbers, and nonexperts are as important as experts. When current reality is accurately apprehended, we can see that we are all enfolded into health care, albeit differently in different roles. Moreover, everyone can see who is included and benefits from health care, who is excluded, and why.

Current reality can be misrepresented by claiming that the current state of affairs is better or worse than it actually is. It can also be misrepresented by withholding, spinning, and doctoring information and by denying the validity of what others have described. Feeling confused about or being punished for telling the truth are signs that the current reality is being misrepresented.

Because it is our habit to discount current reality, being in the moment is something we need to practice. When current reality has not been cultivated, novel information is automatically perceived as a threat. For example, the automatic response to information about a global budget is disbelief. A global budget is in direct opposition to the orthodox beliefs that regulation is bad and market excesses will correct themselves.

Furthermore, the more novel information detracts from the self-serving interests and privileges of those with the knowledge power, the more likely the novel information will be publicly discounted or its validity denied. It is not uncommon for special interest groups to mislead, misdirect, and misinform the public. Examples abound, including the pharmaceutical industry's paying "Flo" to advocate keeping the government out of her medicine cabinet. Another common discounting of reality is seen in stories about the long waiting periods for elective surgeries in Britain that fail to mention the British population's better health status. Even most pharmaceutical advertisements are misleading. Their potent images subtly implant the notion that youth, virility, and wealth come from their pills. In contrast, it's a well-kept secret that in real dollars, Americans' state, local, and federal tax dollars together contribute as much money toward the U.S. health care system as many European governments spend on national health programs that cover their entire population.

Publicly, it is relatively easy to discount current reality. With the blurring of the line dividing editorial content and advertising, it is easy to present only one side of the story, to have unfavorable stories pulled, to attack through negative advertising, and to engage in expensive public relations infomercials. Privately, the discounting of public reality is usually personal. If the information is perceived as too threatening, it is not uncommon to kill the messenger—not literally, of course, but by labeling messengers as sick or as cynics, by firing them, by excluding them from decision-making committees, and by destroying their credibility.

EITHER/OR THINKING

Historically, those who have argued loudest for the status quo—physicians, insurers, and, more recently, the pharmaceutical industry—have resisted changing their minds. They have understood that new feedback loops and the generation of a more holistic health care system would alter their profits and their privileges. To maintain the status quo, these powerful stakeholders take advantage of popular beliefs about health care: that health equals good biomedical care; that science and economics are morally neutral; that market forces can control costs; that government intervention is bad; and that health is a personal commodity, not a social good.

It is not surprising that people attempt to keep things as they are, for fear they will lose what they have. In his book *Not All of Us Are Saints: A Doctor's Journey with the Poor*, David Hilfiker, M.D., speaks poignantly about the effects of fear:

If a compassionate response, in addition, demands of me any redistribution of my wealth, power, or prestige, or if it reveals a vision of a different society in which I am not among the "haves," the temptation to withdraw becomes overwhelming. Is it surprising that, for us who are well-off, numbness so easily replaces compassion as the "natural" response to suffering?[6]

Either/or thinking sets up opposition, generates enemies, and fosters fear. When we are engaged in either/or thinking, we see things as mine or not mine. Unable to see relationships, we see others as competitors. We have no reason to share, or trust there is enough for everyone, or even learn from one another. Even when cooperation among peers is needed to get more goods, our alliances are unstable, formed among independent selves. The greatest fears regarding health care reform have to do with the distribution of resources. Where will the money come from? How will the dollars be distributed? Who decides? Can I trust them to include me? And, spoken more privately, Why should I pay for my neighbor's care when I don't find him or her worthy?

Either/or thinking is a potent method for blocking novel information because it denies interdependence and limits our options: We either compete or control. On one hand, we can't see that a competitor may have resources to share or something to teach us. On the other, we can control what we already know.

In a society that considers surprises as poor planning and a loss of managerial control, letting in novel information or letting something novel emerge is unbearably frightening. Few things make us more insecure than the unknown, more anxious than our own awkwardness with the unfamiliar, and more fearful than our vulnerability to loss. Not trusting change, we seek to keep things as they are for fear we'll lose what we have. It seems safer to preserve the status quo.

NUMBNESS

Fear makes people numb. People who are numb cannot feel. Because numbness is usually mistaken for objectivity, people who are numb are often described as living in their heads. Objectivity has to do with the quantification of things and mathematical calculations, such as drug dosages and returns on investment. When overplayed, objectivity reinforces numbness. By implying a scientific, measured, or value-neutral response, objectivity obscures the motives behind the decisions people make while sanitizing the effects those decisions have on the lives of others.

The status quo is maintained at the expense of feelings. Despite the fact that reasoning and feelings are inextricably linked, objectivity discounts feelings and reinforces control and competition, diminishing people's sensitivity toward one another as a result. We have become inured to other people's suffering, and to our own.

How we feel—or don't feel—about others serves as a mirror for our lives. Our inability to perceive suffering means that we are disconnected from one another, that there is no We. It also means that our heads are disconnected from our hearts; unable to feel, we can't see our own interior world. We lose sight of the tender, vulnerable feelings of love, respect, and caring that form healthy bonds among human beings, for they are eclipsed by our needs to control and compete.

DEFENSIVE ROUTINES

When feelings are discounted, reality is perceived as out there, in the material world. The denial of feelings is a way we deny our interior world. Denying our interior world is how we avoid seeing information about ourselves that doesn't fit with our self-image. Our self-image is the story we tell ourselves about who we are and why we are the way we are. It is our public face, so to speak, but our self-image is not all of who we really are.

Chris Argyris claims that we have developed a skilled incompetence at not knowing all of who we are.[7] We have lost our ability to be real. At an early age, we are programmed to protect our self-image but to conceal that we are doing so. Some of the ways we protect our self-image include wrapping ourselves in political correctness, finding fault, judging others, being overly responsible, sticking to our own kind, limiting our conversations to those we like, and excluding those who are not like us. Referring to the behaviors as "defensive routines," Argyris summarizes them in three categories: blaming, controlling, and withdrawing.

To protect the status quo, we collude with one another's defensive routines: I don't have to tell you any information about myself that compromises my self-image, and I won't ask you any embarrassing questions, either. The problem is, just as an eye needs a mirror to see itself, I understand myself in relation to you. When I am too afraid, ashamed, or apathetic to talk with you accurately about the effect your behavior has on me, or when you are too numb to hear me, I am no longer real to you, nor are you real to me. The relationship itself is unhealthy.

This is a reciprocal hermetic seal. It's a game I play with you to delude myself, so that I don't have to see all of who I am. This perverse skill at protecting one's self-image is built into our social roles. For example, everyone is familiar with the rule of good manners "If you can't say anything nice, don't say anything at all." Doctors and patients quickly learn what information the other is willing to hear. The result is that, in bureaucratic and hierarchical organizations such as health care, secrets are kept, and real problems and difficult information don't easily flow up or down the chain of command. The payoff of this skill is personal, however: I can pursue my self-interests without taking into account the effect my actions have on you.

DISOWNING OUR SHADOWS

Conditioned to identify with our self-image the desirable aspects of our personality, we disown the traits that are unacceptable to our self-image. Desirable doesn't signify good or bad, or effective or ineffective; desirable merely refers to the parts of us we have learned to accept. For instance, imagine making two lists. One list is the attributes you admire in others; the other contains the traits you dislike in others.

Psychologists say that both lists are of traits we ourselves possess, as in the cliché "if you spot it, you got it"; although we usually think of ourselves as being either too good or too bad to claim them. Typically, many of the attributes are positive and negative aspects of the same coin. For example, being responsible is the flip side of controlling. In other words, the attributes are not inherently good or bad, but depend upon the context in which they are displayed.

The attributes we see in others but don't immediately recognize as our own Jungians refer to as our shadow. Considered outside of us, shadows are the attributes we don't claim but project onto others. Shadows indicate where our inner world is poorly integrated; however, shadows also represent resources we don't claim.

When we don't claim all of who we are, several things happen. First, we tend to overplay the attributes we accept; thus overplayed, the attributes become our greatest weakness. For instance, when it is overplayed, caring for others becomes being taken advantage of. Second, not able to see that the outer world is a reflection of our inner world is terribly confusing. We can't differentiate between what's mine and what is not mine. As a result, we either blame others for sabotaging our efforts, attempt to control or "fix" them, or withdraw, fearing for our safety. Third, we underplay our potential. For example, someone who disavows responsibility will have trouble becoming self-reliant. Finally, rather than acting from the current reality, we react. Operating on automatic pilot, we reinforce the status quo and unconsciously reinforce the very behaviors that are harming us.

RE-FORMING THE SELF

Unpacking our self-protective behavior brings us to the root difficulty facing health care reform. Our behavior reinforces the nested hierarchy's modern structure, and the structure reinforces our behavior. With modern concepts incorporated into the self, health care, and the market economy, the tendency to preserve the status quo is very strong indeed, as if three layers of armor protect the health care system. It is this mutual enfolding that makes health care reform so very difficult. In fact, to re-form health care is to re-form the whole hierarchy. To change one is to change them all. The dilemma is that health care reform literally involves feeling safe enough to change our minds, to embrace a holistic rather than a modern perception of the world.

WE ARE WHAT WE THINK

The parable called "The Tragedy of the Commons" can be seen as a metaphor for health care and the fear of not protecting our self-interest. It describes an aggregate of shepherds who graze their sheep on a common pasture. Each shepherd knows that it is in his self-interest to increase the size of his herd, because each additional animal increases his profit, while the damage done to the pasture is shared by everyone. Eventually, growth becomes unsustainable. The pasture is overgrazed, the sheep don't fatten, and the profits to each shepherd begin to drop. By the time the shepherds realize their problem, it is too late to save the pasture.

The moral of the story is that the whole sustains the parts, as in our goldfish bowl metaphor. However, there are other lessons to be drawn from this parable. One is, selfishness pays off, at least in the short run. When the pasture does run out of grass, the losers are those shepherds who have been conscientious, who have done their part to maintain the integrity of the whole. In contrast, those who have grazed the most sheep end up with the most profits. They have more resources and can move to new and better pastures, if there are any. The final lesson is that it is not enough for a few shepherds to see the problem. The problem can't be solved until enough shepherds—what chemists would call a critical mass—act together for the common good.

"The Tragedy of the Commons" is also a metaphor for human thought. The lessons of the parable illustrate how deeply we, as individual human beings, have incorporated modernity's exemplars into our selves. Because of our penchant for objectivity, systems have acquired a life of their own. Having disconnected the observer from the observed and forgetting that the things (Its) we make are ours, inspired by human thought and animated by human hands, the systems control us. Directly and indirectly, these Its shape, sanction, and control our behavior, telling us what to do and rationalizing who is worthy of care.

The danger is not in the utility of objects; objects like nutritious food, clean water, and medicine make life easier and more comfortable. The danger is in forgetting that our rules, roles, and rewards are our own creations. Then, we automatically surrender our decision-making powers to It and, ironically, legitimize that surrender by saying, "The computer won't let me," or "I'm just following the rules."

We are, as S. I. Hayakawa says, "'object-minded' and not 'relation-minded,'"[8] even when we know being selfish is ultimately harmful. We are blinded by modernity, confused by mine versus not-mine, and unable to see the whole of relationships and interdependence. The parable's tragic message is, the habit of shortsighted self-interest is difficult to break. We have become perversely skillful at not seeing the whole.

CHAPTER 8

Compassion

The art of medicine is rooted in the heart. If the heart is false, you will
be a false physician; if the heart is just, you will be a true physician.
Paracelsus

SEEING THE WHOLE

We ended the preceding chapter on a tragic note: that we have become perversely skillful at not seeing the whole. Paradoxically, by unpacking the
nested hierarchy of systems and exposing the ways we have become skillful at repudiating novel information, we caught sight of the whole. We saw
that the whole elephant, metaphorically speaking, is more complex than
our favorite part. By seeing the whole, we transcended modern exemplars;
yesterday's thinking no longer enthralls us. Our thinking has evolved. We
know that we know: the limitations of modern concepts are clearly perceived only in the clarifying presence of new (postmodern) concepts.

A CALL TO BE WHOLE

Intuitively, we know the universe is whole, that it is not separated into
independent parts. The health care crisis is a call to heal what thought has
fractured. Health care's troubles, and our own, arise because, using Ken
Wilber's terminology, we *think* that I, We, and It are disconnected.
Ineluctably, each is a distinct and vital part of the whole, but by itself, each
is broken. Communities and technology both arise from thought, and our
sense of self occurs only in relation to other people and the things we
make. Our troubles arise because thinking that the parts are separate fos-

ters a kind of blindness and numbness to suffering and to the political and moral consequences of our selfish actions.

The health care crisis is a call to be whole: to trust ourselves to change, to embrace a holistic perspective; to see relationships and interdependence; to remember we are connected on the outside to one another and to the things we make (I, We, and It); and to integrate mind, body, and spirit on the inside. To heal health care is to heal our selves.

THE CHOICE POINT

The irony of health care reform is that we can no longer perceive health care as an independent It, totally external to us. Health care is a reflection of human thought. Ideally, health care should represent the best of our thinking, for how we care for others reflects the meaning we give to the preciousness of being human.

At one time, beginning roughly in 1900 and cresting about 1970, the modern health care system did represent the best of human thought. However, the fact that the U.S. health care system ranks first in costs and thirty-seventh in keeping people healthy indicates we need to rethink health care. The system is neither efficient nor effective. It is costly, 43 million Americans are without insurance, population health issues fall through its cracks, and the holistic set of services needed to care for people with chronic and life-threatening conditions is neither integrated nor among its covered benefits.

By now, it should be clear that modern answers to the four questions, What is health, What is care, How much is enough, and Who is responsible? are destined to further destabilize an already dysfunctional system. Moreover, as the step-down influence of the worldview and the market economy on health care is now visible, it is also clear that economic changes applied to health care—in the absence of a balancing loop between health care and the market economy—are not only futile but brutally effect access and quality.

Finally, by sorting through the layers of thought and layers of systems, we have discovered what is internal and what is external to me. We have seen that systemic structure and human behavior are largely mutually reinforcing. This is the choice point. We can continue to delude ourselves, thinking it safer to preserve the status quo, or we can choose to transcend the seeming safety of the known, the familiar, and the status quo to allow something novel to emerge, knowing that we, too, will be changed by a process whose outcome none of us can predict with 100 percent surety.

IT TAKES A VILLAGE...

We know it takes a village to raise a child. It takes a community to reform the health care system. Community means that We is seen, as well as I and It. There is a reserve of social capital, in other words. It's a community endeavor, because re-forming health care entails the incorporation of novel information and sharing resources.

In systems language, health care reform means changing boundaries and adding new feedback loops—a challenge, but doable, nevertheless. The full challenge, however, is more complex. Health care reform also depends on the incorporation of novel, or postmodern, concepts. (Simply put, the term *postmodern* is interchangeable with the terms *relation-minded* and *holistic*.) The incorporation of postmodern concepts means that our thinking has evolved. It does not mean that modern concepts are passé. The body's biochemistry will always act according to the laws of science, and gravity will continue to keep our feet on the ground. It does mean that we will learn to see things differently, more holistically. To return to our Russian doll analogy, incorporating postmodern concepts means that we have enveloped the first four dolls (illustrated in Figure 2.1)—self, health care, market economy, and modern worldview—with a larger fifth doll, the postmodern worldview. It also means that because of the internal consistency requirement, for health care to incorporate holistic concepts, all the other systems in the nested hierarchy must incorporate holistic concepts as well.

When there is internal consistency, meaning is aligned. In terms of health care, aligned meaning signifies congruent answers to the questions What is health, What is care, How much is enough, and Who is responsible? In Flood's language, efficiency, effectiveness, and fairness are coherent with meaning. Where there is coherence, we feel connected to one another and the things we make. When meaning is aligned, people understand and trust one another.

We are back to the fact that people must change for their systems to change. And in any change process, there is a place called the transition zone where old rules, roles, and rewards no longer work but new ways of behaving have not yet been codified or become obvious or taken for granted. The transition zone is similar to the moment when the trapeze artist lets go of the bar behind and hasn't yet firmly grasped the bar in front. It's a place where good intentions often collapse, for we are vulnerable, individually and as stakeholder groups. If we are to trust ourselves to change, we depend on the support of others. Hence, it takes a community to re-form health care.

OUR FRACTURED WORLD

Although it takes a community to re-form health care, the current reality is that health care is an amalgam of disparate parts. It is a loosely held confederation of various delivery systems, financing methodologies, and regulatory agencies and a competitive network of patients, providers, payers, purchasers, purveyors, and politicians. Each has a different view of health care, a view shaped by different regulations, technology, traditions, experiences, beliefs, values, and goals.

Health care's complexity is compounded by the fact that for decades, purchasers, payers, and providers have generally limited their conversations to include only their own kind or a few elite experts. Limiting cross-fertilization of information, cliquishness is a major contributor to health care's inertia. Because of their differences, each group has a different view of health care and its problems; consequently, each group's solution historically has been at the others' expense. Therefore, trust among the stakeholders is not high, having been eroded by the self-serving interests and privileges given to those with the knowledge power.

WE NEED TO TALK

Simply put, the health care system is too large, too complex, and involves too many disparate groups for one group to have all the answers. We need to talk. We create, reflect, and reproduce the health care system through myriad private and public conversations about sickness, aging, death, health, and care. What we choose to bring together or hold apart is influenced by our conversations. Through our conversations, we decide what to do, defend our behavior and our decisions, and define ourselves.

Significant conversations have moral, political, and economic consequences. Who gets invited to the table, what is said, what is discussable and nondiscussable, the questions that are asked and not asked, and what gets heard all either reflect and reproduce the status quo or compel our thinking to evolve.

The health care system we have today is the accrual of at least 300 years of modern conversation, a conversation limited to those with expert knowledge. In contrast, true reform cannot be anything other than a diverse community activity. All of health care's stakeholders are needed at the table, including competitors, colleagues, patients, and the disenfranchised.

Talking together lets us experience what others are feeling, bringing us in contact with one another's suffering and letting us see what the others see. What one person or one stakeholder group may see as an either/or choice, a diverse group will see as a continuum of choices. Here, differences in education, gender, socioeconomic status, regulations, technology, traditions, experiences, beliefs, values, and goals for health care are assets rather than liabilities. They are assets because as much as differences signify the variations in how each of us sees and reproduces our world, differences also represent other ways to see the present moment and, therefore, different ways to negotiate our world, collectively and individually.

A PUBLIC AND A PRIVATE EXPERIENCE

While diversity brings novel information into the system, in actuality the information enters the system through human mouths, is heard by human ears, and is animated by human hands—person by person. It follows, then, that health care reform is both a public and a private experience, governed by the principles of internal consistency and critical mass. To put it bluntly, in order for the health care system to re-form, a critical mass of I's need to re-form as well.

Thus, the phrase "We need to talk" implies a special kind of conversation, one that is very much like the hero's journey, for we are setting out to re-form, or heal, the health care system. While the classical hero's journey was essentially personal, in this conversation, called *dialogue*, healing is occurring on two levels simultaneously: the public and the private.

DIALOGUE: A HOLISTIC CONVERSATION

Dialogue is a kind of mindful conversation; a communal sharing of experiences; a public airing of thoughts, emotions, meanings, and purposes. We reconnect with thought, and in the process we see the condition of minds, for our minds—the lenses through which we see the world—are seen only in reflection. Just as mirrors reflect our biological eyes, the conversations we have with other people reflect the condition of our minds.

William Isaacs,[1] a research director and dialogue facilitator, explains that dialogue is a reflective learning process, one that draws on the work of many, including the philosopher Martin Buber, the psychologist Patrick DeMare, the biologist Francisco J. Varela, and the physicist David Bohm. Dialogue is based on the premise that, generally speaking, all aspects of our society—including our sense of self—are manifestations of thought.

Briefly, dialogue is a way to see and transcend yesterday's thinking that has become so taken-for-granted that it is now invisible, yet that exacerbates health care's precariousness. Unlike discussion and debate, which are conversational methods designed to pound and cut apart, dialogue's usefulness lies in its ability to expose and reconnect us with the thought that spawned the tool, rule, or self-image. In the process, compassion and insight replace competition and defensive routines as the bonds of our relationships.

To overcome any group's tendency to engage in "group think" and keep the nonnegotiables and nondiscussables off of the table, dialogue requires a diverse group of from twenty to forty people. The advantage of a large, diverse group is that its members simply don't know enough about one another to collude in the game of self-protection. Because dialogue takes people beyond the level of individual images and other conversation barriers, it is a conversation that cuts through noble certitudes and cherished self-images, stops automatic-pilot behavior, and exposes us to the effects our actions have on other people's lives.

Dialogue is a hero's journey taken collectively, and like all hero's journeys it is a healing journey. If, during the course of the conversation, meaning has been aligned, purposes defined, roles clarified, goals established, or coherent action has taken place, a connection is formed at a deeper, truer level. We are more integrated, more fully human. As a result, we are freer to create something new and fresh.

HEALING IS THE HERO'S JOURNEY

The hero's journey is a fitting metaphor for health care reform. It is the classic healing journey, often used by patients to describe how they have learned to be whole in the face of chronic and life-threatening sicknesses. In the traditional journey, the hero is compelled to wander through a foreign and frightening abyss in a search for something healing. Traveling alone, the hero encounters helpers along the way. They help the hero slay the dragon, answer the riddles, befriend the heinous, and eventually they provide the hero with a healing potion. If the hero is successful, he or she returns home transformed and resumes his or her worldly business with a more holistic perspective.

The journey involves four stages described in the classic work of Joseph Campbell, *The Hero with a Thousand Faces*.[2] Briefly, the stages begin with a call to change: The signs and symptoms and the suffering can no longer be ignored. When the call to change can no longer be ignored, the second stage of the journey is begun. Some kind of threshold or point of no return has been crossed; it is both an initiation and a death, for the familiar is either dying or receding. In the third stage, the hero encounters the foreign, or the "trials of the road." This is a process of purification involving such things as temptation, betrayal, grief, and forgiveness. Eventually, the hero is given a boon, typically wisdom, which must be passed on to others. Finally, in the fourth stage, the hero returns home reborn; transformed, he resumes his worldly business in new and wiser ways.

In comparison, dialogue, which is a public journey, has no heroes per se, for everyone engaged in the conversation eventually cycles through all three roles: dragon, helper, and hero. Because dialogue is a public journey, the four stages represent the four orders of change taking place in the group. In dialogue language, the group is represented by the term *container*. Container refers to conveyance and to the action of the group. Because action happens in the container, the container needs to be strong enough to contain the action. The container is where we discover that we are the hero, the helper, *and* the dragon, where metaphorical dragons are slain (novel information is no longer repudiated); and it is from the container that we emerge reborn, if the boon is granted.

Isaacs describes the four stages as (1) instability *of* the container, (2) instability *in* the container, (3) inquiry in the container, and (4) creativity in the container. It is instructive to look at each of the four stages of dialogue separately. Although dialogue is presented on paper as a linear process, in actuality, dialogue is a recursive process. In other words, the more the journey unfolds, the more clearly we understand the past and see the reason for the journey.

INSTABILITY OF THE CONTAINER

When any group of people comes together to draw up plans to improve a large system, such as health care, each is wearing a pair of lenses ground according to his or her experiences, prejudices, feelings, emotions, assumptions, values, and beliefs. What each sees is his or her truth. Instability of the container refers to these disparate truths. Participants are like the fabled blind men and the elephant; each sees what he or she is hanging on to but is unable to see what the others are seeing.

In this stage, for instance, deliberations are begun without clarifying or exposing each person's understanding of the meaning of health or the purpose of health care. Those in the conversation simply know that something is wrong and needs to be fixed. Furthermore, deliberations are begun with only a superficial awareness of the needs, desires, expectations, values, and beliefs of the others.

As the group deliberates, it reaches a choice point. The group can continue to formulate adaptive fixes, or it can recognize that it is time for something new to emerge. For example, the group can recognize that today's cost, quality, and access problems exceed health care's range of adaptability, or it can continue imposing piecemeal changes. Like the traditional hero, the group can either answer the call to dialogue or resist the call.

If the group does not understand that something new is trying to emerge, it will resist the call. Intuiting that stepping over the threshold signifies loss, the group will also resist the call if it fears that the cure is worse than the disease. In other words, resistance is a defensive strategy to avoid suffering (although it makes suffering worse), for our unconscious minds hold the delusion that pushing back against whatever is causing us to suffer will make it go away. In this stage, resistance generally manifests as a rush to fix the visible broken part; misrepresenting the data to show that the situation is worse or better than it actually is; claiming what we want is already here; or proclaiming that if others would stop being negative and conform to standards, the problem would be solved.

While some groups don't have the capacity to answer the call, some are willing and able to cross the threshold. As Isaacs says, "this is the moment dialogue confronts its first crisis: the need for the members to look at the group as an entity including themselves as observers and observed, instead of merely 'trying to understand each other' or reach a 'decision that everyone can live with.' "[3]

Answering the call is largely an act of faith. Because the group is an aggregate of independent individuals, each can only assume that the others are equally committed, willing to endure the unknown, and willing to help one another generate what is best for the nation's health. Once they are committed, the second stage of the journey has begun.

INSTABILITY IN THE CONTAINER

Every significant change is preceded by some force that disrupts the status quo. In chemical reactions, for instance, the application of additional energy ruptures the electron bonds of the original molecule, dislodging the molecule from its energy trough and destroying its equilibrium. Illness is a comparable disrupter. Illness unravels familiar roles, goals, and values of the patient and leaves him or her to suffer a terrifying sense of vulnerability. Instability in the container refers to similar losses and feelings of vulnerability and disorganization. The container becomes a crucible for suffering. The familiar has lost its center; artifice and secrets are exposed and stripped away. While some may feel replete with the richness of all possibilities, most engaged in the conversation are sorely tried as they struggle with feelings of confusion and loss. Suffering is the order of the day.

This stage requires that the thoughts, emotions, and perceptions that created the experience be named, be owned by the speaker, and be suspended for public view and reflection. All the thoughts and emotions that are kept below the surface in polite and politically correct conversations are exposed. The conversation reveals health care's underlying incoherence; that is, the misalignment of purpose, effectiveness, efficiency, and fairness and the thought that sponsors the misalignment. The conversation also exposes the myriad inconsistent and incongruent perceptions regarding each of the four elements that generate the health care system. We get to see what others see as they describe their images of health, care, enough, and responsible. This is a dicey place to be! The hero has located the dragons.

A strong container is needed to contain the chaos. It is time for the helpers to step forward. A container's strength depends upon a number of conditions, including the skillfulness of the facilitator, the emotional maturity of the group's members, and the group's ability to distinguish among layers of thought. This refers to unpacking the nested hierarchy and noticing what is being rejected and why. In other words, what part of the nested hierarchy is activating our behavior, causing us to block novel information? Are we acting out of our job role, our socioeconomic status, out of a worldview hardwired into our nervous system, or out of something more personal like fear and selfishness?

Another important condition is the group's commitment to Jurgen Habermas's validity claims:[4]

1. The speaker must tell the truth, i.e., the facts are accurately described, as are the thoughts, feelings, and emotions evoked by the facts.

2. The speaker expresses him- or herself truthfully so the listener can believe what he or she hears and can accept the speaker as trustworthy.

3. The speaker must express information in a way that the listener can accept what is said.

4. The speaker and the listener have to *want* to understand each other. Understanding implies intimacy and equality. In other words, subordination/domination is not operative.

Emotional maturity is key if the group's members are to avoid confusing the dragons with the helpers. Emotional maturity refers to the members' capacity to tolerate vulnerability, ambiguity, and anomie. Mature people have the capacity to model vulnerability by telling their own truth and to accept the emotional and intellectual tension that is experienced when the sources of fragmentation are surfaced. Because they understand that the external mirrors their intrapsychic state, they have empathy for the heinous instead of blame. Instead of seeking revenge, they have concern for one another's welfare. Instead of needing to control, they are curious. Instead of withdrawing, they have the capacity to remain engaged even when nothing seems to hold.

For example, even though a global budget can control costs and give all Americans access to a predetermined level of care, it doesn't come preassembled and ready to be plugged in. So that we don't continue to recreate the same old thing dressed up in new clothes, the stage instability in the container exposes health care's underlying incoherence and its normally invisible operating rules.

It also illuminates health care's roles, rules, and rewards, which are the supporting beams of any system. Because any role and its concomitant rules and rewards are the intersection of the system with the individual, it is challenging not to take these conversations personally. At this stage, the group will surface long-standing economic and power struggles among the dominant stakeholders (physicians, hospital administrators, and insurance executives, for instance); deep animosity and professional jealousies (such as between doctors and nurses); and fear and blame for health care's high costs and ineffectiveness.

Feeling the Wounds

Instability in the container is marked by feelings of anger and chaos, which are anathema to people who see themselves as caring and in control. Anger signals that boundaries have been broken. Generally, we assume that anger originates in the individual, but that is too easy. Placing all the focus on the individual conceals the influence the other systems in the nested hierarchy have on the individual's behavior.

The architect Christopher Alexander eloquently speaks to the influence of nested contexts in the design of buildings. According to Alexander, buildings that are configured to fit the environment and the needs of those who use them generate a kind of quality that livens and animates the people who live and work inside them. The quality is mutually reinforcing. We have all felt it; hospital administrators refer to this as a healing environment. When buildings are designed with what Alexander calls "structural contradictions," however, the buildings bleed off vital human energy. Even in the design of buildings, one can't escape the influence of politics and economics.[5]

Most health care organizations are riddled with structural contradictions: roles, rules, and rewards that are at cross-purposes to one another. A typical example is an organization that espouses teamwork but rewards employees according to a merit pay system. Howard Waitzkin, in his book *The Second Sickness: Contradictions of Capitalist Healthcare*, exposes many of health care's structural contradictions, such as downstream medical treatment for upstream environmental toxins and the costly expansion of coronary care units without proof of their effectiveness.[6] In other words, health care is not an isolated system but is structured according to beliefs emanating from the larger political and economic contexts, which means that health care cannot change without similar changes occurring in these larger contexts.

Structural contradictions tend to wound the people enfolded into the system. Poignant examples of structural wounding involve notions regarding responsibility and self. For instance, when overplayed, responsibility results in being used, neurotic caretaking, and controlling behavior; underplayed, however, leads to being overly dependent and under-self-reliant. Moreover, modernity's championing of the self leads to selfish behavior among those who hold the knowledge power. The elite status of experts has led to the separation of operations and planning, the separation of delivery and finance of care, and command-and-control management and has set up paternalistic doctor-patient relationships. The assumption that the individual is responsible for outcomes has also colored our ideas about who is worthy of health care, concealing the effect the economy, education, geography, and history have on a person's health and access to health care. Perhaps the deepest wound of all is the belief that there is no need for the government or society to meddle: The We has dropped out of sight.

The dragon is a symbol for our wounds. Our notions about roles and responsibility are internalized, or incorporated into our self-image. When our notions cause us to overplay or underplay any attribute of our self-image, we are acting out of our wounds, so to speak. To generalize, marginalized and disenfranchised people are plagued by feelings of self-doubt, hopelessness, helplessness, and anger; those who have the knowledge power feel that they have to have all of the answers and be in control.

In dialogue, these internal thoughts and feelings surface for public view. No longer numb, this is a painful place to be. For the most part, the sensation is expressed as anger, for boundaries are coming down. Generally speaking, caretaking professionals habitually deny their anger, and most people who have made it to positions of power have developed a kind of sophistication that allows them to deny any sense of helplessness and suppress feelings of impotence and rage or feelings of fear toward those who are different. It is a social norm to keep anger in the shadow. When suddenly exposed, anger morphs into a heinous creature. Although awfully personal, the raw feelings that emerge during this stage of the inquiry are wounds we carry for society. In this stage of the journey, we are like medical students in training. Not yet skillful, we are often symptomatic for everything we treat as we learn to care for the wounded. Hence the need for experienced helpers, or facilitators.

The fragmentation and the structural contradictions are shards of thought. When the shards finally cut into our awareness, we feel their jagged edges. In other words, we begin to feel our own brokenness. No one can accurately claim to be an innocent victim. At this stage, if compassion, truthfulness, and trustworthiness are not actively cultivated, or if people need to hang on to old beliefs and behaviors like shields, the container quickly collapses. The participants, in mythical terms, have confused helpers with dragons. However, if the group can ask itself, "What is society having the individual experience because of his or her role?" then individual versus systemic versus worldview operating rules are untangled, and it is possible to reconnect thought and behavior to the appropriate context.

INQUIRY IN THE CONTAINER

Although suffering continues until integrity is restored, a compassionate response indicates that the container has held. Inquiry in the container is a sign of compassion, which means the group is sensitive to the various ways the conversation is affecting everyone. This stage is similar to the fifth of Stephen Covey's habits of highly effective people: "Seek first to understand, then to be understood."[7]

This stage signifies that the conversation has changed. Conversations are how we are formed and informed; they are the primary ways we know who we are. Thus, a change in the quality of the conversation indicates that we, too, are changing. It is a tandem process—either we change and the conversation changes, or the conversation changes and we change. The breakdown occurs if one process gets ahead of the other. Then, we lose our bearings and don't know how to understand the experience. Inquiry in the container means that change is happening; healing is beginning to occur.

Compassion

Compassion means to suffer or experience with—to actually feel another's weal and woe. Compassion is more than pity, sympathy, or mercy; they contain elements of patronization. But compassion connotes a sense of shared humanity, an active regard for the other's good, and recognition that the relationship is reciprocal. Thus compassion supplants the temptation to blame, control, withdraw, or take advantage of the sufferer. Compassion transforms the fiery crucible into a healing space in which the sufferer gives voice to his or her experience and needs.

Regardless of what induced the suffering, a compassionate response entails three stages. The first stage is witnessing the other's distress. This is simply being present in the midst of overwhelming chaos to show the sufferer that he matters and won't be abandoned to the forces that are destroying his life as he knows it. The second stage is giving the sufferer permission to lament, to tell his story, give voice to his experience and all the rawness it entails. As the helper inquires into the sufferer's experience, frightening, and confusing feelings give way to words: The collage of thoughts, emotions, beliefs, and conditioning the sufferer has lived by is exposed. Once the hardwired conditioning melts in the clear light of awareness, the person knows himself more fully. Grasping and rejection cease; the dragons are slain. Finally, if what is needed is present, the person has the freedom to embrace new values and new meaning. He returns home more whole.

To be compassionate, people need the courage to be real, to embrace their own humanness, their imperfections and inadequacies. Knowing that the imperfections seen in others are also reflections of their own condition, the compassionate have developed equanimity toward that which is false, ugly, threatening, or frightening. Equanimity is not resignation, but a kind of peace that comes from knowing that all opposites eventually balance in one still point. Having learned firsthand to trust that it is safe to surrender the illusion of the small, separate self, the compassionate are able to accept the sufferer for who she is, challenge her to embrace her potential fullness, yet protect her through the difficult passages where she is vulnerable to destruction.

Long known as integral to healing and once the mainstay of biomedical care, compassion is as critical to health care reform as it is to patient care.

Just as chronic disease alters a patient's self-image and autonomy, the integration of new feedback loops will alter some aspects of the traditional roles, and privileges each group of stakeholders now enjoys.

In dialogue, roles are often reversed, and compassion is offered by whoever has the "firmer handhold on the climb." For example, a forty-year-old woman with stage IV breast cancer—acutely attuned to the signals of her body, well informed about the poor probability for five-year survival and the debilitating side effects of treatment—commits medical heresy. She opts to forgo aggressive treatment and chooses palliative care instead. To eschew treatment flies in the face of her doctor's training. Withholding permission to do what he can to prolong the patient's life challenges his clinical competency and stirs up fears about his own mortality. To walk this edge takes incredible compassion. The patient cannot abandon the physician; she needs his expertise for palliative care. Instead, the patient must accept the doctor as he is, for she knows that the beliefs about aggressive care and fear of death are not hers. She has no need to make him wrong regarding his beliefs about life-prolonging high-tech care, and because she faces her nearing death with courage and equanimity, she thus protects him where he is vulnerable.

Those are rare times, when the physician realizes the patient's compassion for his plight. Feeling her compassion forms an opening for the provider to see beliefs he has taken for granted. He begins to see what she has known all along: that death is a natural part of life, and that caring is not synonymous with curing. That she depends on him to manage her pain, provide information, and help tell her family what is happening to her body releases him from guilt and his own false expectations. If he is lucky, his traditional stance softens, and he begins to see new possibilities for the questions What is health? What is care? Who is responsible? and How much is enough? Freed from biomedicine's tradition of having to have all the answers, this physician, paradoxically, has more choices regarding the ways he engages with his patients. Suddenly, his own suffering ceases.

Reconciliation

The integration of new feedback loops will disrupt existing boundaries, beliefs, and behaviors now held fast by each stakeholder group. For this reason, the cultivation of compassion, which is cultivated with Habermas's validity claims, is essential to health care reform. If compassion is not present, the stakeholders feel forced to continue defending themselves and the status quo. They will keep the system out there and hang on to traditional responsibilities. The risks are simply far too great when others can't be depended on to sacrifice personal autonomy for the good of the whole or in any other way to transcend the status quo.

When compassion is cultivated and people feel understood, they feel safe enough to befriend their own brokenness. Unlike knowledge, which implies separation from and mastery of the object, understanding involves intimacy and equality between self and object. Akin to the German word *kennen* and the Greek word *gnosis*, understanding implies a personal acquaintance with the object—usually, but not always, another human being. Moreover, because understanding entails nonjudgmental acceptance, people begin to embrace aspects of themselves they have disavowed and projected onto others. In other words, people begin to connect their thinking with its manifestations. Internally, mind, body, and spirit are reunited; and externally, the three-way connection among the selves, other people, and the health care system emerges into plain sight.

Thus it is safe to embrace new identities and responsibilities, to share resources for the good of the whole, to collaborate rather than compete. This kind of reconnection is also known as reconciliation or redemption. Although reconciliation refers to rebuilding a fractured relationship, the significance of repair work is that people can trust that intimacy and equality will hold. For example, given that the existing system fosters economic competition, imagine the trust it will take for stakeholders to assume new responsibilities and share resources. Imagine the amount of reconciliation it will take for those who now fall into the have and have-not categories to trust each other.

Reconciliation is the boon granted by the fraternal twins of forgiveness and grief. Briefly, grief is the public acknowledgment that we have lost something precious to us. Loss may range from petty neuroses and noble certitudes to position, money, real estate, and even life itself. Grief involves mourning; acknowledging rather than resisting the loss; and actually feeling the pain, anger, dread, helplessness, and so forth as they arise. Grief does not mean wallowing in these feelings, nor does it mean self-pity or blame. We can grieve unskillfully, that is, we can resist the loss. Like a closed fist, this only furthers our isolation and separateness. Conversely, we can be skillful and perceive the loss as having our hand opened so that we can hold on to something new.

Forgiveness, on the other hand, refers to ceasing to feel resentment. It is about finding meaning and equanimity in the midst of the trials others put us through. Phillip Moffitt reminds us "forgiveness is not about helplessly accepting, giving up, surrendering to defeat, being weak, or avoiding the cost of justice."[8] Forgiveness is not about bargaining or being weak, which simply creates more doormats; nor is forgiveness about resistance. Resistance, a defensive strategy, hardens our hearts and makes suffering worse. Instead, forgiveness is the practice of opening our hearts *and* holding others accountable; or of finding compassion "while you act in the world to correct that wrong and try to prevent it from happening again," as Moffitt says.[9]

Reconciliation is another word for healing. What once was broken has been reunited. While reconciliation neither means perfection or that the past has been restored, reconciliation signifies a new or transcendent relationship. In other words, the heroes are transformed and can resume their worldly business with a more holistic perspective.

Reconciliation happens on several levels. By slaying the dragons, the hero has integrated mind, body, and spirit on the inside and has integrated I, We, and It on the outside. In the context of dialogue, healing is opening to new knowledge and understanding; healing is what dialogue refers to as creativity.

CREATIVITY IN THE CONTAINER

Finally, if a diverse group is able to follow a thread of ever-more-profound inquiry, then thought, its manifestation, and human behavior are reunited. This reunion sparks such clarity of understanding that a spontaneous and radical realignment of meaning occurs. Thought has been transformed. A higher level of integration emerges from this insight. Human beings can embrace their differences as well as their similarities. Opposites are balanced. This is true creativity. From this new thinking comes a different way to behave. The way is so clearly defined that there is no confusion, nothing to debate; only one new way to act.

The alchemy of dialogue is that it understands life to be a two-way street. Human beings are connected: to one another, to the things they make, and to the biosphere. By caring for others, we care for ourselves. And, although the transition zone is fraught with hazards, the disruption of the status quo is the only gateway to something more profoundly intact.

Basically, the route of dialogue follows a recursive four-step process. The process is not linear, but it does unfold one step at a time. We can't skip steps and jump right to creativity. To skip to creativity, to say "Can't we just work together; let's just make a plan," indicates that the status quo is still intact. The preconceived pictures still exist; the differences have not been accounted for. Suffering, compassion, and respect have been denied. With the heart of the matter silenced, creativity is stillborn. At best, the result is a revision of the status quo; at worst, health care slides a little closer to the abyss.

THE HEALER ARCHETYPE

In the classical hero's journey, the helper, the hero, and the dragon are three different entities; similarly, in clinical medicine, the physician, the patient, and the remedy are different entities. In dialogue, however, everyone has an opportunity to be the helper because each person cycles through the dragon, hero, and helper roles. In fact, the outcome of dialogue largely depends upon the presence and skillfulness of the helpers, a role that embodies the healer archetype. Thus it is useful to health care reform that we explore the healer archetype.

Archetypes, according to Carl Jung, are deep, abiding patterns in the human psyche that remain powerful and present over time.[10] For the ancients, they were the gods and goddesses literally interacting with human beings. Now representing prototypical qualities, their names have carried forward: *Asclepius,* the god of medicine, and *Hygeia,* the goddess of health. The archetype is always whole and does not change, although the concept, names, and symbolic images vary according to time and place. Because the archetype personifies the quintessential, the archetype's power lies in its ability to bring about what the conscious mind alone is incapable of either understanding or achieving.

Although the roles of the physician in clinical medicine and the helper in dialogue are both healer roles, there are important distinctions between them. The physician and patient are independent entities and the relationship is essentially mechanical, because the physician is not changed by the relationship and the remedy is external to both the patient and the physician. Accordingly, the physician's power lies in his technical competency. In contrast, the helper in dialogue is more like the archetypal healer: Wounded, being wounded, and healing are three equally potent powers of the archetypal healer.[11] The dialogic relationship is essentially organic and the helper's competencies lie in his ability to point out and activate healing powers that the other unknowingly possesses. Ideally, both the patient and helper are healed by the relationship.

Briefly, healing is the symbolic act of dying and the birthing of a new, more integrated whole. (Healing is always more than returning to the status quo.) Healing is precipitated by a wound that symbolizes the destabilizing of the status quo. The wound also symbolizes a doorway into a new, more integrated whole. The stability of the emerging whole usually requires two remedies, support and sacrifice. (Support means that a missing element is supplied from the outside; sacrifice entails surrendering or reframing what is worn out or toxic.) Paradoxically, the archetypal healer doesn't "fix" the problem; instead, through his wounds and healing powers, the healer activates the healing powers of the patient. That is to say, the archetypal healer is a catalyst, an agent that lends its energy to initiate and speed up the reaction but that is not changed by the process.

In dialogue, helpers embody the archetypal powers: wounding, being wounded, and healing. The three powers make the helper role in dialogue indeed dicey. Being wounded and healing are easy to understand because a system and its stakeholders are mutually enfolded. Dysfunctional systems foster dysfunctional roles and impair relationships, which is wounding to stakeholders. Conversely, for the system to be healed, the relationships among its stakeholders must be healed as well, which requires personal changes in the behavior and thoughts of each of the stakeholders.

The power to wound, however, signifies the misuse of power. Helpers who overestimate their power wound themselves. Self-wounding occurs when a healer goes beyond his or her catalytic capacity. This happens when the system's capacity to push back, or another stakeholder's power, is stronger than the healer's power. For instance, imagine stakeholders dialoguing about the redistribution of economic resources. As their anxiety increases, trust evaporates and the group polarizes. If the group blames the convener for letting things get out of hand, that person will carry the untrustworthiness for the group. This attitude may follow the convener and he may be excluded from further financial decisions.

Self-wounding also occurs when the healer uses up his or her own life force in the change process. This is a rescue fantasy, which nurses call burnout. Moreover, hard-to-heal issues and recalcitrant stakeholder groups can easily become a battleground where the issue or the stakeholder group becomes something to be defeated and dominated. Such behavior on the helper's part deactivates the healing power of the other stakeholders, which turns off the system's capacity to heal.

Conversely, helpers who misuse their power—such as the power to raise prices and to deselect patients—further wound other stakeholders. In both cases, power is used to protect present rights and privileges, but the effect on the patient is diminished quality and more costly access to health care.

In contrast, recalcitrant stakeholders can override the healing power of the helper by abnegating their responsibilities and by scapegoating. Abnegating their own power to heal, these stakeholders blame the helper for unresolved problems while surreptitiously enjoying secondary gains. Here, self-reliance is in short supply and helper burnout is very high. Scapegoating occurs when a stakeholder group insists that the problem is external and refuses to redistribute its resources or reconcile its relationships. In fairy tales, the princess won't kiss the frog.

The healer archetype mediates the mystery of wounding, being wounded, and healing. The doctor-patient relationship is always under the influence of these three archetypal powers, and those who are aware of its forces receive its blessings. Similarly, health care's stakeholders' relationships are also under the influence of these three potent archetypal powers. Dialogue is premised on their awareness; the conversation evolves to the extent those engaged in the conversation are willing to do the hard work of personal healing and systemic role reform. Of course, human beings will always be less than the archetypal ideal. We are mortals with limited gifts and skills, broken by our own fears and frailties, and never sure that our perception of mystery is congruent with its nature.

LEVELS OF READINESS

The purpose of dialogue is to heal what thought has fractured. Dialogue, which tacks between the personal and the public, is the contemporary hero's journey taken en masse.

In dialogue, healing is personal and public. Healing is the deeper integration or balancing of parts perceived as outside by our unconscious mind. Healing is also described as leveraging diversity,[12] or by saying that the intelligence of the whole is greater than the sum of the parts.[13] The challenge is that each part is required to give up some of its autonomy in order for the ensemble to function intelligently. In other words, dialogue occurs to the extent that each person is able to commit to befriending brokenness in the pursuit of becoming relation minded.

However powerful and valuable dialogue may be, it is not for everyone. It is tempting to enroll the entire community because health care's turmoil spins on the stakeholders' competitive behavior. Not everyone has the capacity to tolerate the anomie, awkwardness, confusion, and vulnerability such profound change requires. Not everyone has a yearning to be whole.

Readiness to dialogue begins with the cultivation of trust and trustworthiness, for they are largely unavailable to groups that have a history of competitive behavior. A high tolerance for error is also important. New knowledge is always an act of betrayal, giving away a noble certitude or a cherished self-image, for instance. Because information usually enters the container raw and incomplete, the tolerance of the group tested. Not all groups can smooth out and rework the jagged edges of partial truths and incomplete ideas. This is a soul-searching process that often feels like taking one step forward and three steps back, for trust and trustworthiness must be rebuilt every time something new enters the container.

Generally, it is wise to start small and go slowly, for the taxes of reconciliation are high. This is the time to practice and learn dialogue with those who are willing to examine their own motivation and who are committed to balancing their own needs with others. Even here, though, the healing is profound.

THE PARADOX OF WHOLENESS

The heart of health care reform is to connect the pieces, to heal what thought has fractured, and to befriend our brokenness. Inside the heart, however, lies a paradox: We cannot escape our brokenness. Death, disease, and old age will always be with us; enveloped inside our own skin, we will never be one with our neighbor. The paradox to healing, then, lies in befriending our brokenness: accepting the limits of the material world, releasing our habit of projecting our unworthiness on to others, and embracing the parts of ourselves we feel are unworthy of care.

Health care reform is not about designing the perfect system, or one that is free of flaws or satisfies every need of everyone. Perfection is an unachievable ideal. Instead, health care reform is about integrating what thought has fractured and creating a system that produces what is best for the nation's health. Basically, reform is about changing our minds and opening our hearts; we already know the high-leverage changes to boundaries and relationships that can lead to a predetermined level of care for all citizens at a predetermined price.

CHAPTER 9

We

...the path of healing leads not back whence we have come, but ahead, toward a new beginning.

Marc Ian Barasch[1]

TRUSTING OURSELVES TO CHANGE

As though we were traveling along a Möbius strip, we return to our starting point. Health care is about many things and can be understood from multiple points of view—economic, scientific, ethical, legal, and even spiritual. But in the end, health care is about people. It is a network of human relationships that people have designed. Health care can never be more effective, more efficient, or fairer than the image in its designers' minds. That image, of course, is the designers' meaning of health.

In many ways, health care reform is like a chronic disease. On one hand, the health care system will always be adjusting to perturbations, for we can assume that in the future newer worldviews will envelope our postmodern understanding of the world. On the other hand, because health care reform and chronic diseases both unravel familiar relationships and self-images, we can learn to rebind and strengthen relationships, evoking new levels of intimacy; or we can let the relationships fray or fracture.

The parallel between personal illness and health care reform is clear and instructive: We are vulnerable to the actions of others. Although the media is replete with stories of families and even whole communities "joining hands and hearts to help an ailing member," much more often the sick are treated like Job, whose friends "not only refuse him real comfort, but even castigate him as he sits helpless in the dust."[2]

Health care reform is similar. By definition, reform is the reassignment of resources and the reformatting of relationships, radically altering traditional roles, rules, responsibilities, rights, and privileges.

This is a transition zone, a place of chaos where nothing is taken for granted as the old no longer applies. In this rapidly shifting confluence of frightening and unfamiliar conditions, the requisite new habits for each stakeholder are very fragile, indeed. In this zone, to which health care reform will repeatedly return us, we are most literally at one another's mercy. When roles and resources change, significant parts of our self-image change as well, leaving us feeling bereft, as though we had been thrown to the wolves.

Transition—gaining fluency, dignity, and comfort with new levels of resources, new responsibilities, and a new self-image—depends upon mutual and reciprocal help: We ↔ I. As every hospital chaplain knows, we need others to guide us in our confused and traumatized condition, to help us make decisions that will provide the maximum use of our potential. Furthermore, in times of chaos, we need others to sustain us: to console us, to help us consolidate our resources, and to help us endure and eventually transcend a destabilizing situation.

If we default to selfish needs to control and to old, competitive habits to take advantage of the chaos for personal gain, then, of course, trust will be abrogated and reform will collapse. But if we can hold the intent to heal the health care system by becoming more whole ourselves, we can join our hands and hearts to support and protect one another as we develop new habits and new ways of being. Then, knowing that we all are included, each one can trust that he or she will survive the personal changes health care reform will exact.

AN OPEN HEART

In contrast to U.S. society, some indigenous societies see a reciprocal relationship between disease in the personal body and the social body. They see a mutual and reciprocal relationship between individual sickness and society. For example, individuals who break a taboo or are envious can be the source of social disharmony; reciprocally, social disharmony can cause sickness in individuals. In such societies, caring for the whole community is as important as caring for an individual member.

Among the Jul'hoansi of the Kalahari Desert, sickness and well being have profound personal and interpersonal implications. According to the anthropologist Richard Katz and his colleagues, the concept of "heart" is significant to Jul'hoansi understanding of health and healing. A "happy heart" is a state of love and indicates both a sense of personal wholeness and the harmonious connections with others necessary for social cohesion.

A happy heart is an "open heart." Open hearts are essential to the activation of nǀom, the spiritual energy that is the basis of Juǀʼhoan healing. An open heart also signifies courage to engage with nǀom, trust in the community's support, dedication to serving the community, and "passion to sustain the healer's journey despite periods of doubt and 'failure.'"[3] Although the tribe's healers control and direct the nǀom, nǀom can't be hoarded or used for personal gains. Instead, the more it is used, the more abundant and more valuable the healing energy becomes.

At its core, healing is a transformation of consciousness, which the healers experience most of all. The transformation of consciousness enables healers to channel nǀom to cure sickness, resolve issues dividing the group, and affirm spiritual cohesion. Because the energy works on physical, psychological, social, and spiritual planes, healing occurs on multiple levels. By connecting people together in harmony, the individual's worth is affirmed and the group's awareness of behaviors essential to maintaining the welfare of the whole is elevated.

Unfortunately, Americans don't have methods for healing the whole. Even though we talk about sick buildings, failing systems, and an unraveling social fabric, sickness is still treated one person at a time. Both metaphorically and scientifically speaking, heart work is significant to health care reform. First, we have repeatedly seen the significance of an open heart regarding the health status of both individuals and populations. Love, esteem, and respect—synonyms for an open heart—are the health-producing ingredients inherent to intimate relationships and the social determinants of health. Moreover, love, esteem, and respect affect the health status of individuals and whole populations. Second, as with Juǀʼhoansi healers, an open heart—with its concomitant association of courage, trust, dedication, and passion—is vital to sharing resources and power and to sustaining stakeholders through the periods of doubt, failure, and grief that will be encountered while health care is re-formed.

THE COURAGE TO CHANGE

Those who engage in the challenging work of health care reform are healers in the truest sense of the word: They know that they embody the wound and the remedy. Healer/reformers know that health care itself is sick. It costs too much; excludes too many; fragments care; burns out health care workers; separates mind, body, and spirit; and reduces the community to an aggregate of independent individuals. Such fragmentation prevents the various stakeholder groups from realizing the moral and material consequences their actions have on others.

Throughout the United States, small groups of intrepid healers are experimenting with a variety of new ways to organize, deliver, and pay for health care. They clearly see the impact the dysfunctional system has on their communities, their patients, and themselves, and they have the courage to generate something different. Aware of the benefits and the pain inherent in the modern health care system, their desire is not to start all over or reinvent the wheel, but to experiment, re-forming that piece of health care that is within their sphere of influence. Because they understand that re-form is a group process that health care is comprised of relationships, and that human relationships hang by the thin thread of conversation, these courageous healers have spent a lot of time talking, forging partnerships, and building collaborative relationship and thus have discharged the inertia of the status quo. A representative sampling follows.

NEW BEGINNINGS

Wellspring for Women

When a provider acknowledges his or her own suffering, something profoundly transformative begins. Despite telling her patients to listen to their bodies, CeCe Huffnagle was not heeding her own advice. A nurse practitioner and director for the women's center of a large, wealthy suburban hospital, she felt her job was becoming more about public relations than about caring for the women who sought her expertise regarding women's health issues. There were not enough hours in the day to meet the marketing department's demands plus the demands of her own heart. Work and its frustrations were always on her mind, and she began having chest pains and problems with her blood pressure.

With the help of friends, Huffnagle disentangled the hospital's goals from her personal goals. She saw that one of the hospital's goals was to survive in a highly competitive market, which meant that the women's center was a means to achieve brand recognition. In contrast, her personal wish was to provide care for women in the perimenopausal years of their lives. Accepting the differences, she knew her heart soared when she was caring for individual women and their health concerns.

Huffnagle decided to risk going into private practice, a novel endeavor for a nurse practitioner. Partnering with nurse practitioner Carol Dalton, she formed a holistic health center, Wellspring for Women. Although based on the concepts of Christiann Northrup, M.D., Wellspring is unique. Huffnagle and Dalton work for themselves, not for a physician. Patients are billed directly because third-party reimbursement is not accepted, but the nurse practitioners follow the insurance industry's billing procedures so that patients can collect whatever their policies allow.

At Wellspring, the mind/body/spirit is cared for as one ensemble. Because disease in the body may be as much about dis-ease in the mind or spirit, treatment at Wellspring is not limited to drugs. In fact, Huffnagle and Dalton are knowledgeable about both biomedicine and alternative practices, so they can mix and match treatments. Moreover, in contrast to the typical short doctor's appointment, appointments at Wellspring generally last a full hour. Addressing the health concerns of perimenopausal women takes time because changes in libido and bone density, incontinence, depression, and so forth affect lifestyle as well as physiology. Perceiving their patients as more than physical bodies, the nurse practitioners spend much of their time helping their patients take stock of their lives. These nurse practitioners understand that a patient's habits and activities, her family and job, her dreams and disappointments, are as important to her health as are lab results and estrogen replacement therapy.

Aware of their limitations as nurse practitioners, they do not hesitate to refer. Most significantly, they share their time as well as their expertise. Instead of expeditiously reducing the patient to a broken body part, Huffnagle and Dalton make the time to develop a trusting relation, share information, and answer questions. They make time for the patient's mind, body, and spirit to be cared for as a whole.

The creation of Wellspring for Women illustrates that human beings and their systems are mutually enfolded. One affects the other; one can't change without the other's changing. This is not to say that Huffnagle's transformation changed the health care system. But Huffnagle changed. When she was no longer able to function with integrity within the confines that corporate health care set for nurse practitioners, she acknowledged her suffering and pursued her own healing. Consequently, health care changed as well, albeit in a very small way.

Wellspring for Women fills a need for integrated care. Patients are satisfied with Wellspring's blend of alternative and traditional care. Huffnagle and Dalton are happy, for they are delivering health care in a way that is true to their hearts. Patients are satisfied as well. In fact, Huffnagle and Dalton have a full practice and are looking for another partner. Their success is being replicated as Wellspring has become a model for other nurse practitioners. In 1998, the Holistic Health Nurses Association recognized Wellspring as an exemplar of care.

Kaiser-Permanente of Northern California Redesigns Chronic Disease Care

Even though the death rate for chronic disease became greater than the death rate for infectious disease around 1925, the health care system didn't change its practice habits. So what does an insurance company do when 25 percent of its subscribers have some type of chronic disease?

Millions of Americans now live with asthma, diabetes, heart disease, arthritis, back pain, visual and hearing impairments, and other chronic conditions. While these conditions are rarely cured, biomedicine typically manages them in ways that emphasize diagnostic and curative interventions. Organized prior to the rise in the incidence of chronic diseases, biomedicine was never intended to "strengthen and support the abilities of patients and families to self-manage chronic disease"[4] or to help patients manage the psychological and social effects of chronic disease. Unfortunately, this gap has significant human and economic costs to the patient and society.

A wide range of studies has shown that when patients with chronic diseases receive psychosocial support, are taught self-management skills, and are routinely monitored, the patients do better. That is, the patients feel better, follow their doctors' orders better, are more active, miss fewer days of work, and are more involved with their family and social groups. Moreover, patients have fewer symptoms, have a greater sense of control over their disease, and are more satisfied with their medical care.[5]

Aware of these studies, a small group of intrepid leaders at Kaiser-Permanente of Northern California decided to address the unique needs of the chronically ill. Their long-term goal was to create a delivery system that partnered with these patients. A bold experiment for health care, it was made possible by Kaiser's founding principle of keeping people healthy and its status as an integrated system. Because doctors, hospital staff, and payers work for the same company, issues such as turf and profit, which usually derail a mixed group of stakeholders before it gets started, were not insurmountable. This made it easier to rewire long-standing roles and reporting structures and to modify the way information was shared and used.

For three years, doctors, nurses, allied health professionals, health educators, administrators, project managers, and data analysts met. Talking about their dreams, their fears, and their turf; taking the best from the bits and pieces of research; and sustained by their desire to integrate all three components—psychosocial support, self-management skills, and routine monitoring—they gradually hammered out an astronomical number of details.

Theirs is a radical design, establishing a partnership among patients, physicians, and allied health. Patients are not passive consumers but are active participants in their own care. Medical needs are dealt with proactively rather than by having patients wait for the traditional office appointments after their symptoms have appeared. Physicians attend to problems identified from the patient's perspective as well as to the traditional biological signs and symptoms. Finally, patients are taught self-management skills and provided with routine monitoring and are supported in making behavioral changes.

The prototype is now being tested on patients with asthma, congestive heart failure, and diabetes, so it is too early to evaluate the effectiveness of the design. If patients are enrolled in group appointments and support groups, will they share information, learn from, support, and encourage one another? If patients are routinely monitored, will they follow the doctor's orders, seek help before their symptoms become acute, and not blame the physician if they don't get well? If patients are taught self-management skills, will they monitor their symptoms and take appropriate action? If patients become healthier, will they require fewer services?

Moreover, if the design does effectively support chronic disease management, what are the long-term outcomes? Will patients report they feel better, have fewer sick days, miss fewer days of work, participate in family and civic responsibilities, and use fewer health care resources? It is a bold experiment, for the redesign tacitly reforms the patients' expectations of health care, and reforms the providers' and patients' expectations of each other.

A Local Solution to a National Problem

Despite a variety of government incentives, most rural areas are underserved. It takes a special kind of physician to practice in isolation, to be away from peers, to be always on call, and to not have ready access to subspecialists and high-tech support for serious emergencies. Besides, physicians' families typically want better cultural activities, shopping, and schools than rural areas offer. The long hours, the lack of amenities, and the difficulties in earning a reasonable income make it difficult for small, rural towns to attract and keep physicians.

When two of its four physicians retired in 1984, Burlington, Colorado, began recruiting for two physicians, an intense and disappointing search that was to last more than eight years. Located on the eastern plains of Colorado, Burlington (population 3,055) is a small farming community with a twenty-five-bed hospital, the Kit Carson County Memorial Hospital. The hospital's inability to recruit new physicians was not only medically troublesome, it hurt the town economically. Instead of waiting months for a doctor's appointment, people found it easier to drive thirty miles to Goodland, Kansas, or sixty miles to Denver, where they combined big-city shopping with doctor's appointments. It wasn't just sundries and groceries they bought; some even came home with new cars.

When local reporter John Hudler heard that Sacramento Pimentel and James Perez, two graduates of Burlington High School, were looking for loans to pay for medical school, the recruitment problem was on its way to being solved. Instead of the hospital's continuing to pay for costly searches and coming out empty-handed, why not pay Pimentel's and Perez's medical school tuition? After all, both aspiring physicians grew up in Burlington the sons of Mexican farmworker families; were used to small-town living; and wanted to return to Burlington, to practice where they knew people as friends and neighbors as well as patients.

Harold McArthur, a John Deere contractor, agreed with Hudler. Moreover, McArthur, who is as generous and progressive as he is wise, agreed to pay the tuition for both students. In return, Pimentel and Perez agreed to practice in Burlington one year for every year their tuition was paid. The deal was closed with a handshake.

In January 2000, Pimentel and Perez opened their family practice in a new clinic built for them by the hospital. By all accounts, it's a win-win solution. The doctors' practice is full; all four doctors share call. They like the variety of medical problems, caring for people from birth to death, and having time to know their patients as people with families and jobs. The town likes the new doctors—their bedside manner, that they speak Spanish, and that they make house calls. As Hudler says, the town is delighted.[6] He doesn't understand why other rural communities don't do the same.

Bridging the Mind-Body Split

With a few experimental exceptions, health care still adheres to the mind/body split. Forcing two kinds of problem, two kinds of clinician, two kinds of treatment, and two kinds of covered benefits means that patients must be willing and able to navigate two systems, as neither system talks to the other. Causing clinical ineffectiveness, operational inefficiencies, and financial waste, this arrangement is costly.

Frustrating operational inefficiencies—doctors perpetually behind schedule and a high no-show rate among patients with mental health problems—were the impetus for the staff at Marillac Clinic to integrate medical and mental health into one delivery system. Briefly, Marillac Clinic provides medical, dental, and optical care to about 6,000 poor and uninsured patients living in Grand Junction, Colorado. Fifty-one percent of the patients live on less than $10,000 a year. Approximately 50 percent of the medical patients suffer from depression or anxiety, are victims of crime, or have substance abuse problems that are tightly entwined with their physical problems. When the clinic's providers referred these patients to mental health professionals, however, only two in ten patients showed up for their first appointment. This, the Marillac staff knew, indicated weaknesses in the existing system.

Because Marillac is a small, nonprofit clinic, it was able to integrate mental and medical care quite rapidly. Much as a staff model HMO, Marillac's clinical, operational, and financial functions were already integrated. Providers were either employees or volunteers. Because funding was primarily through donations, grants, and patient fees, services were not determined by insurance rules and regulations. Thus any cost savings would mean more money for patient care.

Searching for a viable model, they settled on collaborative family health care, a proven model that systemically integrates mental and medical care. With help from Larry Mauksch, a professor of family medicine at the University of Washington who spent a year on sabbatical at Marillac, the clinic's staff pursued its goals of taking care of the whole person.

Marillac formed a consortium with four local mental health agencies. In three short years, medical providers were trained to detect and evaluate psychosocial problems as a routine part of the patient's history and physical. With the implementation of interagency referral forms and the sharing of medical and mental health records, the mental health, medical, and social service systems now talk to one another within the consortium. Finally, charitable funds were raised to assure that Marillac patients have access to community mental health services.

In the collaborative model, the patient establishes the focus of his or her care. Together, in a thirty-minute office visit, the medical provider and the patient agree on a treatment plan that addresses not just diabetes or hypertension but also addresses psychosocial conditions, such as using alcohol to relax or worrying about money, that tend to worsen the physical condition.

Because mental health is routinely incorporated into medical care, and because appointments for counseling are made by Marillac's staff, patients are more accepting of mental health care. The numbers bear this out. Nine out of ten patients now show up for their first mental health appointment. Equally important, the number of no-shows and scheduling problems has significantly decreased, leaving more time for Marillac's providers to see more patients.

Anecdotal evidence indicates that patients and medical and mental health providers are pleased with their integrated system. Patients typically feel better and are more satisfied with their care. Providers, too, have fewer frustrations with the system, for they now have a method for sharing information and resources. These results are typical of all collaborative-care initiatives. Still, the Marillac Clinic is unique. It is receiving national attention because it is the only program directed at the uninsured and because it is the first program in which five independent community agencies are partnering with one another to provide health care that bridges the mind/body split.

In May 1999, the consortium was awarded a four-year, $471,000 matching grant from the Robert Wood Johnson Foundation. The monies are received and administered by the clinic. According to executive director Janet K. Cameron, they would be used to hire a full-time case manager and two full-time counselors to pay a part-time substance abuse evaluator and psychiatrist, and to fund support groups for patients with chronic diseases and substance abuse problems.[7]

The consortium planned to use this four-year period to focus on out-come evaluations. Its members hope that the numbers at the end of the grant period will show that Marillac patients used fewer hospital days than they did before, that blood sugar levels for diabetics were more often within normal limits, and that patients suffering from depression reported a better quality of life and fewer disability days. The thought is that by using the collaborative model to improve quality and cut costs, more money will be left over for Marillac to care for more of Grand Junction's uninsured patient population.

Supportive Care of the Dying: A Catholic Coalition for Compassionate Care

In 1994, six Catholic health care systems came together to form Sup-portive Care of the Dying: A Coalition for Compassionate Care. By 1998, this number had grown to fifteen members with health care ministries in forty-eight states. Originating as an alternative to physician-assisted sui-cide, the coalition thought the primary issue was patients' fear of dying in uncontrollable pain. Focus-group research revealed, however, that pain management was just the tip of the iceberg. The deeper issue—the many forms of emotional, economic, and social assistance patients with life-threatening illness need if they are to live fully until they die—is eclipsed by health care's acute-care design and society's belief that life-threatening illness is a medical problem only.

Championing the goal of helping people live fully until they die, the coalition sees itself as an advocate for creating partnerships between the health care system and the community. Now completing their second phase, coalition members are engaged in a variety of projects that include research regarding the information, services, and support needed by patients, their families, and their communities; the develop-ment of models of comprehensive community-based supportive care; and the creation of education programs for professional providers and the community.

One example of a partnership is a medication assistance program for needy patients. By hiring a pharmacy technician to do the paperwork that patients wouldn't or couldn't do, the Providence Health System in Port-land, Oregon, was able to use pharmaceutical indigent programs to obtain more than $350,000 worth of medicine for more than 500 low-income patients. This was more than the $250,000 Providence spent annually on drugs for the indigent.

Another coalition-sponsored project, led by the Archdiocese of Philadel-phia, involves partnerships among health care organizations, health care education programs, and community social services professionals and volunteers. Understanding that living fully occurs in the community, the project focuses on linking health care resources with those of the patient's community. Volunteers may spend time with the dying, relieve family members, and help patients and their families access a variety of community and health services. This is especially important in culturally diverse communities because only the patient's own community can serve as a cultural interpreter for health care services.

Additionally, the coalition has partnered with St. Louis University School of Medicine to study changing physician practices from a disease-centered, biological-problem focus to a more holistic view of care. The redesign encourages physicians to become empathetic listeners and involve their patients in structured support groups oriented toward the spiritual, emotional, and relational aspects of the end of life. It also encourages discussion of the possibility of death as an outcome of illness. Patient participants in this program report greater satisfaction with their physicians' communication and less fear of death.

In its third phase, the coalition will develop strategies and support to replicate and implement the learning from the pilot projects. It will also focus on strengthening the community partnerships where each of the member organizations is present.

The coalition understands that organizations seeking to provide comprehensive health care must go beyond biomedicine's acute-care mentality; involve the community, care for the mind and spirit as well as for the bodies of those with life-threatening illness; and support families, friends, and caregivers, too. As Patrick Cacchione, the coalition's board chairman says, "The road to cultural change is long and often uphill. Yet the needs and the benefits are clear."[8]

A Living Wage

In the service sector, where low-wage jobs are concentrated, living-wage policies are usually anathema. Yet for St. Joseph's Health System, a living-wage policy makes sense on many levels. The philosophy behind the living wage is simple: low-wage earners have the right to live and work with dignity and respect rather than live in poverty. Consequently, pay rates are calculated so that low-tier, full-time wage earners can afford the basic needs of life: housing, food, transportation, and health care.

St. Joseph's Health System, which is owned by the Sisters of St. Joseph's of Orange, has about 22,000 employees in twenty-four hospitals in California, New Mexico, and Texas. The living-wage philosophy fits neatly with the Sisters' core values of justice, excellence, service, and dignity and with the broader Catholic values of social justice. Clearly guided by its values, it is a unique organization, even for Catholic health care. Its living-wage policy was implemented in 1997. While the policy is part of a broader focus on compensation, it is also due to the Sisters' understanding of, in the words of Jack Glaser, director of St. Joseph's Center for Health Care Reform, "the need to change social structures that define us as unjust institutions."[9]

Wages are calculated to keep a one-wage-earner family of four above the poverty level. When first implemented, the policy affected about 25 percent of St. Joseph's workforce. Nurse's aids and dietary, laundry, and housekeeping employees were the most immediately affected. Typically, they are health care's low-wage earners.

Another feature of the compensation policy is a career advancement benefit implemented at the employees' request. Employees who qualify get scholarship money, work reduced hours, and receive full-time pay so they can work while attending school.

Does the living-wage policy benefit the employer? The answer is yes, according to Cindra Syverson, senior vice president of human resources. At St. Joseph's, the employee turnover rate is 5.6 percent lower than the industry standard. In an era of nursing shortages and constant recruitment, the numbers speak for themselves.

HEALTH MEANS WHOLENESS

Since the 1970s, economic and moral forces have shifted the mission of health care away from caring for the needs of sick people to maximizing profits. To maintain the illusion of stability, health care counters its soaring costs with precipitous reductions in access and quality. In this fiercely competitive atmosphere, costs are uncoupled from quality and access. Profits count, not people.

Health means wholeness. The health care crisis is a contemporary call to be whole: to find congruent answers to health care's four elemental questions (What is health, What is care, How much is enough, and Who is responsible?) and concomitantly generate a coherent system in which efficiency, effectiveness, and fairness are aligned with the meaning of health.

Try as we might, we can't change health care's problems without changing the other systems that are parts of health care's nested hierarchy (Figure 9.1). Because the notion that the parts are more important than the whole—which prevents the various stakeholder groups from experiencing the moral and material consequences their actions have on others—and the myriad conflicting images and structural contradictions now destabilizing health care all arise from human thought and are institutionalized in the general social fabric, the healing journey is simultaneously public and private.

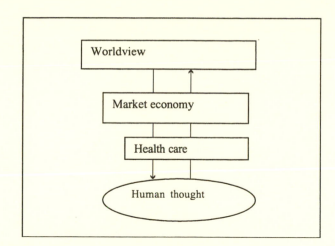

Figure 9.1 The Market Economy and Health Care Are Derived from a Worldview, and All Emerge from Human Thought

To change health care is to change our minds, and to change our minds is to open our hearts. If we hold in our hearts the intent to heal health care by becoming more whole ourselves, dialogue will take us beyond fragmented solutions, beyond consensus, and beyond adaptations of the status quo. Through these conversations, the Cartesian split between spirit and matter reunites, the path between the head and the heart is opened, and relationships are strengthened.

As we come to understand our interrelatedness—system after system, or layer of thought after layer of thought—the whole picture becomes clearer. Two things happen. First, by reconnecting thought with its manifestations, we are reminded that our tools and technology, our laws, our moral codes, and our economic systems are mere manifestations of our thought, and the benefits and pain we cause others by our moral and material choices are revealed. Second, by seeing the layers of thought, we can more clearly discern what is inside and what is outside the self; expose the source of structural contradictions; and identify, among the layers of thought, the actual location of high-leverage opportunities.

To hold the intent to heal is heart work; yet the conversational coin of the heart is infinitely thin, for we can know the other only to the extent we are willing to know ourselves. Still, when we empty our hearts of resentment, greed, and hate, our eyes become clearer. Seeing a bigger picture, what was once an either/or choice becomes a question of balance. We are able to risk wisely, for we understand what choices are ours to make. Able to work in multiple contexts, we understand what we have control over and what we don't. It is an iterative process, one that should support us in the face of re-forming health care.

BUILDING ON THE RUN

Because all systems are interrelated, even the best of plans will always fall short. Our knowledge will always fall short of a full understanding of the entirety of the exquisitely fine-tuned and infinitely interlocking variables of these nested relationships. Some people simply say that we can't know God's mind. To add to the difficulty, all systems are in motion, requiring us to learn to build on the run and to realize that nothing is permanent. All of life is a series of overlapping beginnings and endings. No wonder we want control, to hang on to the familiar, and hope that we can determine the outcome. But by letting go of mechanistic, deterministic thinking, we gain our freedom. We remember from whence we came.

Notes

CHAPTER 1

1. Steuerle, C. E. (1997). The search for adaptable health policy through finance-based reforms. In R. B. Helms (Ed.), *American Health Policy: Critical Issues for Reform.* Washington, D.C.: DAEI Press.

2. Medical bills play big role in bankruptcies. (2000, April 25). *USA Today.* Available: http://www.usatoday.com/life/health/care/lhhca090.htm

3. Reinhart, E. E. (1994). Providing access to healthcare and controlling costs: The universal dilemma. In P. R. Lee & C. L. Estes (Eds.), *The Nation's Health* (4th ed.). Boston: Jones and Bartlett, pp. 263–278.

4. World Health Report 2000. (2000). *Health Systems: Improving Performance.* Geneva, Switzerland. p. 155.

5. Starr, P. (1982). *The Social Transformation of American Medicine.* New York: Basic Books, p. 285.

6. Starr. (1982). *The Social Transformation of American Medicine*, p. 313.

7. Findlay, S., & Miller, J. (1999). *Down a Dangerous Path: The Erosion of Health Insurance Coverage.* National Coalition on Health Care. Available: www.nchc.org/releases/erosion.html

8. Feldstein, P. J. (1998). *The Politics of Health Legislation: An Economic Perspective.* Ann Arbor, MI: Health Administration Press.

9. Budetti, J., Duchon, L., Schoen, K., & Shikles, J. (1999, Fall). "Can't afford to get sick: A reality for millions of working Americans." *The Commonwealth Fund Quarterly.* Available: http://commonwealthfund.org/publicist/quarterly/index.asp

10. Liska, D. (May 1997). *Medicaid Overview.* Available: http://www.urban.org/url.cfm?ID=307044

11. Navarro, V. (1992). Medical history as justification rather than explanation: A critique of Starr's *The Social Transformation of American Medicine.* In V. Navarro (Ed.), *Why the United States Does Not Have a National Health Program.* Amityville, NY: Baywood, p. 42.

12. For more information regarding the influence of class, see Rothman, D. J.(1997). A century of failure: Healthcare reform in America. In P. Conrad (Ed.), *The Sociology of Health and Illness.* New York: St. Martin's Press; and Navarro. (1992). *Why the United States Does Not Have a National Health Program.*

13. Clanham-Clyne, J., Himmelstein, D., & Woodhandler, S. (1995). *The Regional Option for a National Health Program.* Stone Creek, CT: Pamphleteer's Press, p. 43.

14. *Health Spending: The Growing Threat to the Family Budget.* (1991, December). Washington, D.C.: Families USA Foundation.

15. Maxwell, S., Moon, M., & Sega, M. (2000, December). *Growth in Medicare and Out-of-Pocket Spending: Impact on Vulnerable Beneficiaries.* Urban Institute. Available: www.urban.org/health/growth-in-medicare.html

16. Steuerle, C. E. (1997). The search for adaptable health policy through finance-based reforms.

17. Starr, P. (1995, Winter). *What Happened to Healthcare Reform?* Available: http://www.prospect.org/print/v6/20/starr-p.html

18. Budetti, Duchon, Schoen, & Shikles. "Can't afford to get sick."

19. Brandon, R. M., Podhorzer, M., & Pollak, T. H. (1992). Premiums without benefits: Waste and inefficiency in the commercial insurance industry. In V. Navarro (Ed.), *Why the United States Does Not Have a National Health Program.* Amityville, NY: Baywood, pp. 73–90.

20. Feldstein, P. J. (1988). *The Politics of Health Legislation: An Economic Perspective.* Ann Arbor, MI: Health Administration Press.

CHAPTER 2

1. *NPR/Kaiser/Kennedy School Poll on Health Care.* Available: http://www.npr.org/news/specials/healthcarepoll/index.html

2. Senge, P. (1990). *The Fifth Discipline: The Art and Practice of the Learning Organization.* New York: Doubleday.

3. Senge. (1990). *The Fifth Discipline.*

4. Deming, E. W. (1986). *Out of the Crisis.* Cambridge, MA: MIT Press.

5. Berwick, D. (1990). *Curing Health Care: New Strategies for Quality Improvement: A Report on the National Demonstration Project on Quality Improvement in Health Care.* San Francisco: Jossey-Bass.

6. Flood, R. L. (1999). *Rethinking the Fifth Discipline: Learning within the Unknowable.* London: Routledge.

7. Flood. (1999). *Rethinking the Fifth Discipline,* p. 70.

8. Rawls, J. (1971). *A Theory of Justice.* Cambridge, MA: Belknap Press.

9. Bohm, D., & Edwards, M. (1991). *Changing Consciousness.* New York: Harper San Francisco.

10. Wilber, K. (1995). *Sex, Ecology, Spirituality: The Spirit of Evolution.* Boston: Shambhala.

CHAPTER 3

1. *Webster's New World Third Collegiate Dictionary.* (1988). Springfield, MA: Merriam-Webster, Incorporated.

2. Starr, P. (1982). *The Social Transformation of American Medicine.* New York: Basic Books.

3. Brown, E. R. (1979). *Rockefeller Medicine Men: Medicine and Capitalism in America.* Berkeley: University of California Press. p. 122.

4. Brown, E. R. (1976). Public health in imperialism: Early Rockefeller programs at home and abroad. *American Journal of Public Health, 66,* 897–903.

5. http://www.swho.int/about/en.

6. United Nations International Covenant on Economic, Social, and Cultural Rights. (1967). Available: http://www.unhchr.html/menu3/bla_cescr.htm

7. Callahan, D. (1977). Health and society: Some ethical imperatives. In J.H. Knowles (Ed.), *Doing Better and Feeling Worse: Health in the United States.* New York: Norton. p. 26.

8. Rifkin, J. (1995). *The End of Work: The Decline of the Global Labor Force and the Dawn of the Post Market Era.* New York: Putnam, p. 178.

9. Anspaugh, D. J., Hamrick, M.H., &. Rosato F. D. (1997). *Wellness: Concepts and Applications.* St. Louis, MO: Mosby, p. 5.

10. Evans, R. G., & Stoddart, G. L. (1994). Producing health, consuming health care. In R. G. Evans, M. L. Barer, & T. R. Marmor (Eds.), *Why Are Some People Healthy and Others Not? The Determinants of Health of Populations.* New York: Aldine De Gruyter, pp. 27–63.

11. Sontag, S. (1978). *Illness as Metaphor.* New York: Farrar, Straus and Giroux.

12. Spake, A. (1998, December 21). The valley of death. *US News & World Report,* pp. 53–54.

13. Egolf, B., Lasker, J., Wolf, S., & Potvin, L. (1992). Featuring health risks and mortality: The Roseto effect: A 50-year comparison of mortality rates. *American Journal of Public Health, 82*(8), 1089–1092.

14. Evans, R. G., & Stoddart, G. L. (1994). Producing health, consuming health care. In *Why Are Some People Healthy and Others Not? The Determinants of Health of Populations,* p. 43.

15. Milio, N. (1994). The profitization of health promotion. In J.W. Salmon (Ed), *The Corporate Transformation of Health Care: Perspectives & Implications.* Amityville, N.Y.: Baywood, pp. 75–89.

16. Mesa County. *Our Picture of Health.* (1995). Grand Junction, CO: Civic Forum, p. i.

17. *What is population health?* Available: http://www.hc-sc.gc.ca/hppb/phdd/approach/index.html

18. Tarlov, A. R., & St. Peter, R. F. (2000). Introduction. In A. R. Tarlov & R. F. St. Peter (Eds.), *The Society and Population Health Reader: A State and Community Perspective.* New York: New Press, pp. x–xi.

19. *What is population health?* Available: http://www.hc-sc.gc.ca/hppb/phdd/approach/index.html

20. *NPR/Kaiser/Kennedy School Poll on Health Care.* Available: http://www.npr.org/news/specials/healthcarepoll/index.html

21. McKeown, T. (1988). *The Origins of Human Disease.* New York: Blackwell.

22. Susser, M., Hooper, K., & Richman, J. (1983). Society, culture, and health. In D. Mechanic (Ed.), *The Handbook of Health, Health Care and the Health Profession.* New York: Free Press, p. 24.

CHAPTER 4

1. Stein, H. F. (1990). *American Medicine as Culture.* Boulder, CO: Westview Press, p. 41.

2. Kilborn, P. T. (Feb. 1, 1998). Race-health discrepancy persists. *The Denver Post*, p. 2A; Brown, D., & Goldstein, A. (Dec. 4, 1997). Death knocks sooner for D.C.'s black men. *The Washington Post.* p. A01.

3. McKeown, T. (1988). *The Origins of Human Disease.* New York: Blackwell.

4. www.canadian-health-network.ca/1determinants_of_health.html

5. Maslow, A. H. (1968). *Toward a Psychology of Being.* New York: Van Nostrand Reinhold.

6. Cousins, N. (1979). *Anatomy of an Illness as Perceived by the Patient: Reflections on Healing and Regeneration.* New York: Norton.

7. Von Korff, M., Gruman, J., Schaefer J., Curry, S. J., & Wagner, E. H. (1997). Collaborative management of chronic illness. *Annals of Internal Medicine, 127,* 1097–1102.

8. Ornish, D. (1998). *Love and Survival: The Scientific Basis for the Healing Power of Intimacy.* New York: HarperCollins, pp. 2–3.

9. Berkman, L. F., & Syme, S. L. (1979). Social networks, host resistance, and mortality: A nine-year follow-up study of Alameda County residents. *American Journal of Epidemiology, 241,* 186–204.

10. Spiegel, D. (1993). *Living beyond Limits: New Hope and Help for Facing Life-Threatening Illness.* New York: Times Books.

11. Ornish. (1998). *Love and Survival,* pp. 175–186.

12. House, J., Karl, S., Landis, R., & Unberson, D. (1988). Social relationships and health. *Science, 241,* 540–545.

13. Berkman, L. F., & Kawachi, I. (2000). *Social Epidemiology.* New York: Oxford University Press; and Evans, R. G., Barer, M. L., &. Marmor, T. R. (Eds.). (1994). *Why Are Some People Healthy and Others Not? The Determinants of Health of Populations.* New York: Aldine De Gruyter.

14. Bird, S. T., & Bauman, T. E. (1995). The relationship between structural and health services variables and state-level infant mortality in the United States. *American Journal of Public Health, 85,* 26–29.

15. King, G., & Williams, D. R. (1995). Race and health: A multidimensional approach to African-American health. In B. C. Amick S. Levine, A. R. Tarlov, & D. Chapman (Eds.), *Society and Health.* London: Oxford University Press, pp. 93–130.

16. Kilborn, P. (1998, February 1). Race-health discrepancy persists. *Denver Post*, p. 2A.

17. Epstein, H. (1998, July 16). Life and death on the social ladder. *New York Review of Books, 45,* 26–30.

18. Durkheim, E. (1951). *Suicide.* New York: Free Press.

19. Kawachi, I., & Kennedy, B. P. (1999). Health and social cohesion: Why care about income inequality. In I. Kawachi, B. P. Kennedy, & R. G. Wilkinson (Eds.), *The Society and Population Health Reader: Vol. 1. Income Inequality and Health.* (Vol. 1). New York: New Press, pp. 195–210.

20. Miller, S. M. (1995). Thinking strategically about society and health. In B. C. Amick S. Levine, A. R. Tarlov, & D. Chapman (Eds.), *Society and Health,* pp. 342–358.

21. Wilkinson, R. (1999). The culture of inequality. In I. Kawachi, B. P. Kennedy, & R.G. Wilkinson (Eds.), *The Society and Population Health Reader: Vol. 1*, pp. 492–498.

22. Erlich, P. R., & Erlich, A. H. (1991). *Healing the Planet: Strategies for Resolving the Environmental Crisis*. Boston: Addison-Wesley.

23. Patrick, D. L., & Wickler, T. M. (1995). Community and health. In B. C. Amick S. Levine, A. R. Tarlov, & D. Chapman (Eds.), *Society and Health*, pp. 46–92.

24. Byrd, R. C. (1988). Positive therapeutic effects of intercessory prayer in a coronary care unit population. *Southern Journal of Medicine, 81*(7), 6–29.

25. Oxman, T. E., Freedman, D. H., & Manheimer, E. D. (1995). Lack of social participation or religious strength and comfort as risk factors for death after cardiac surgery in the elderly. *Psychosomatic Medicine, 57*(1), 5–15.

26. Oman, D., & Reed, D. (1998). Religion and mortality among the community-dwelling elderly. *American Journal of Public Health, 88*(10), 1469–1475.

27. Personal communication. Ulricke Dettling Kalthofev. (Dec. 2001). Arlington, MA; and Hoover-Kramer, D., Mentgen, J., & Scandrett-Hibden (Eds.). (1996). *Healing Touch: A Resource for Health Care Professionals*. Boston: Delmar.

28. Institute of Medicine, Committee on Quality Health Care in America. (2001). *Crossing the Quality Chasm: A New Health System for the 21st Century*. Washington, D.C.: National Academy Press.

CHAPTER 5

1. Nichols, L. (1998). Health Care Quality at What Cost? Available: http://www.urban.org.url.cfm?ID=306795

2. Fry, J.D., Light, J. R., & Orton, P. (1997). The US health care system. In P. Conrad (Ed.), *The Sociology of Health and Illness: Critical Perspectives* (5th ed.). New York: St. Martin's Press, p. 210.

3. *National Average Wage Index*. Social Security Administration. Available: http://www.ssa.gov/OACT/COLA/AWI.html

4. Fry, Light, Rodnick, & Orton. (1997). The US health care system, p. 210.

5. Woodhandler, S., & Himmelstein, D. U. (1991). The deteriorating administrative efficiency of U.S. health care. *New England Journal of Medicine, 324*, 1253–1258; Woodhandler, S., & Himmelstein, D. U. (1997). Costs of care and administration at for-profit and other hospitals in the U.S. *New England Journal of Medicine, 336*, 769–774.

6. Woodhandler, S., & Himmelstein, D. U. (2002). National health insurance, liberal benefits, conservative spending. *Archives of Internal Medicine, 162*, 973–975.

7. Green, M. (1999, April 12). Regulators may derail Anthem-Blues Linkup. *BestWeek Life/Health*.

8. Heffler, S., Levit, K., Smith, S., Smith, C., Cowan, C., Lazenby, H., & Freeman, M. (2001). Health spending growth up in 1999: Faster growth expected in the future. *Health Affairs, 20*, 193–203.

9. Woodhandler & Himmelstein. (2002). National health insurance, liberal benefits, conservative spending, 973–975.

10. Starr, P. (1994). *The Logic of Health-Care Reform*. New York: Whittle Books, p. 17.

11. Aaron, H.J., & Schwartz, W.B. (1984). *The Painful Prescription: Rationing Hospital Care*. Washington, D.C.: Brookings Institution.

12. WHO issues new healthy life expectancy ratings. (2000, June 4). *World Health Organization.* Available: http://www.who.int/inf-pr-2000/en/p2r000-life. html.

13. Becker, E. (1973). *The Denial of Death.* New York: Free Press, p. 2.

14. Hoover, D. R., Cantor, J., Kumar, R., Sambamoorthi, U., & Crystal, S. (2000, November 14). Elderly Medicare and non-Medicare end of life expenditures in the MCBS from 1992–1996. *The 128th Annual Meeting of the American Public Health Association.* Available: http://apha.confex.com/apha/128am/techprogram/paper _6182.htm

15. Maicki, H.W. (2000, Summer) G..a..p..s in the end-of-life care. *Supportive Voice.* Available: http://www.careofdying.org/SV/PUBSART.ASP?ISSUE+SV00 SU&ARTICLE=D

16. Mairs, N. (2001). *A Troubled Guest: Life and Death Stories.* Boston: Beacon Press, p. 10.

17. Strosberg, M. A., Wiener, J. M., Baker, R., & Fein, I. A. (1992). *Rationing America's Medical Care: The Oregon Plan and Beyond.* Washington, D.C.: Brookings Institution.

18. Day, K. (2000, January 17). Your money or your health. *Washington Post National Weekly Edition,* p. 21.

19. Blendon, R. J. (1988). What should be done about the uninsured poor? *JAMA, 260,* 3176–3177.

20. Schneider, E. C., Zaslavsky, A. M., & Epstein, A. M. (2002). Racial disparities in the quality of care for enrollees in Medicare managed care. *JAMA, 287,* 1288–1294.

21. Bach, P., Cramer, L. D., Warren, J. L., & Begg, C. B. (1999). Racial differences in the treatment of early-stage lung cancer. *New England Journal of Medicine, 341,* 1198–1205.

22. Whittle, J., Conigliaro, J., Good, C. G., & Lofgren, R. P. (1993). Racial differences in the use of invasive cardiovascular procedures in the Department of Veterans Affairs Medical System. *New England Journal of Medicine, 329,* 621–627.

23. Hadley, J., Steinberg, E. P., & Feder, J. (1991). Comparison of uninsured and privately insured hospital patients. *JAMA, 265,* 374–379.

24. Greenberg, W. (1998). *The Health Care Marketplace.* New York: Springer, p. 43.

25. Leape, L. L. (1992). Unnecessary surgery. *Annual Review of Public Health, 13,* 363–383.

26. Chassin, M. R., Galvin, R. W., & National Roundtable on Health Care Quality. (1998). The urgent need to improve health care quality. *JAMA, 280,* 1000–1005.

27. Chassin, M. R., Galvin, R. W., & National Roundtable on Health Care Quality. (1998). The urgent need to improve health care quality. *JAMA, 280,* 1000–1005.

28. McPherson, K., Wennberg, J. E., Hovind, O. B., & Clifford, P. (1982). Small-area variations in the use of common surgical procedures: An international comparison of New England, England, and Norway. *New England Journal of Medicine, 307,* 1310–1314.

29. Adams, M. E., McCall, N. T., Gray, D. T., Ozra, M. J., & Chalmers, T. C. (1992). Economic analysis in randomized control trials. *Medical Care, 30,* pp. 231–243.

30. Von Korff, M., Gruman, J., Schaefer, J., Curry, S., & Wagner, E. H. (1997). Collaborative management of chronic illness. *Annals of Internal Medicine, 127,* 1097–1102.

31. AARP. (1992). *9 Ways to Get the Most from Your Managed Care Plan.* (Publication No. CARE5546(1297).D16615.) Washington, D.C.: AARP.

32. Ornish, D. (1990). *Dr. Dean Ornish's Program for Reversing Heart Disease.* New York: Random House.

CHAPTER 6

1. Flood, R. L. (1999). *Rethinking the Fifth Discipline: Learning within the Unknown.* New York: Routledge, p. 116.

2. Flood. *Rethinking the Fifth Discipline,* p. 116.

3. Parsons, T. (1981). Definitions of health and illness in the light of American values and social structure. In A.L. Caplan, H. T. Engelhardt, & J. J. McCartney (Eds.), *Concepts of Health and Disease: Interdisciplinary Perspectives.* Reading, MA: Addison-Wesley, pp. 57–82.

4. *Workers' compensation benefits decline as a percentage of wages for seven years in a row.* (2001, May 22). Available: http://www.nasi.org/publications2763/ publications_show.htm?doc_id+57955

5. Michaels, D. (1988). Waiting for the body count: Corporate decision making and bladder cancer in the U.S. dye industry. *Medical Anthropology Quarterly, 2*(3), 215–232.

6. MacLennan, C. A. (1988). From accident to crash: The auto industry and the Politics of injury. *Medical Anthropology Quarterly, 2*(3), 233–250.

7. Waitzkin, H. (1983). *The Second Sickness: Contradictions of Capitalist Health Care.* New York: Free Press, pp. 3–43.

8. Research study by economists Mary Merva and Richard Fowles of the University of Utah. (1995). In J. Rifkin. *The End of Work: The Decline of the Global Labor Force and the Dawn of the Post Market Era.* New York: Putnam, p. 178.

9. Dembe, A.E. (1996). *Occupation and Disease: How Social Factors Affect the Conception of Work-Related Disorders.* New Haven, CT: Yale University Press, p. 257.

10. Spake, A. (1998, December 21) The valley of death: Researchers probe a mysterious plague of heart disease. *US News & World Report,* pp. 53–54.

11. Gussow, Z. (1989). *Leprosy, Racism, and Public Health: Social Policy in Chronic Disease Control.* Boulder, CO: Westview Press, pp. 8–9.

12. Hoffer, T., Haywood, R., Greenfield S., Wagner, E., Kaplan S., & Manning W. (1998). Unreliability of individual physician's "report cards" for assessing the costs and quality of care of chronic disease. *JAMA, 281,* 2098–2105.

13. Frank, A.W. (1995). *The Wounded Storyteller: Body, Illness, and Ethics.* Chicago: University of Chicago Press.

14. Taylor, F.W. (1967). *The Principles of Scientific Management.* New York: Norton.

15. *About chronic disease.* Center for Chronic Disease Prevention and Health Promotion. Available: http://www.cdc.gov/nccdphp/about.htm

16. Institute of Medicine. (2001). *Crossing the Quality Chasm: A New Health System for the Twenty-first Century.* Washington, D.C.: National Academy Press.

17. *Medicaring: A new model for end-of-life care.* Available: http://www. asaging.org/am/cia2/mediCaring.html

18. Institute of Medicine. (2001). *Crossing the Quality Chasm.*

19. Bringewatt, R. (2001). Making a business case for high quality chronic illness care. *Health Affairs, 20,* 59–60.

20. Knowles, J.H. (1997). The responsibility of the individual. In P. Conrad (Ed.), *The Sociology of Health and Illness: Critical Perspectives,* (5th ed.). New York: St. Martin's Press, pp. 382–392.

21. Mechanic, D. (1994). *Inescapable Decisions: The Imperatives of Health Reform.* New Brunswick, NJ: Transaction, p. 108.

22. Morreim, E.H. (1995). *Balancing Act: The New Medical Ethics of Medicine's New Economics.* Washington, D.C.: Georgetown University Press, p. 2.

23. Fry, J., Light, D., Rodnick, J., & Orton, P. (1997). The US health care system. In Conrad, *The Sociology of Health and Illness,* pp. 206–214.

24. Morriem, *Balancing Act,* pp. 86; 85–98.

25. *Health Insurance—Universal Coverage.* (2002, January 31). Available: http://www.stateaction.org/issues/healthcare/uhi/index.cfm

26. *KFF State Health Facts Online: 50 State Comparisons: Population Distribution by Insurance.* Available: http://statehealthfacts.kff.org/cgi-bin/healthfacts.cgi?action =compare&category=Health+Co

27. National Academy Press. (2001). *Coverage Matters: Insurance and Health Care,* p. 11. Available: http://books.nap.edu/html/coveragematters

28. Senge, P. (1990). *The Fifth Discipline: The Art and Practice of the Learning Organization.* New York: Doubleday, pp. 27–54.

29. Hayakawa, S.I. "The Revision of Vision." In G. Kepes. (1995). *The Language of Vision.* New York: Dover, p. 10.

CHAPTER 7

1. NPR/Kaiser/Kennedy School Poll on Health Care. Available: http://www.npr.org/news/specials/healthcarepoll/index.html

2. Dellums, R. V., et al. (1977). *Josephine Butler United States Health Service Act* (H.R. 1374). Washington, D.C.: Government Printing Office.

3. Institute of Medicine. (2001). *Crossing the Quality Chasm: A New Health System for the Twenty-first Century.* Washington, D.C.: National Academy Press.

4. http://www.gwu.edu/~cicd/medicaring/NewMediCaring1298.html

5. Canadian Health Network. (2001, November 26). Available: http://www.canadian-health-network.ca

6. Hilfiker, D. (1994). *Not All of Us Are Saints: A Doctor's Journey with the Poor.* New York: Hill & Wang, p. 179.

7. Argyris, C. (1986, September). Skilled incompetence. *Harvard Business Review.*

8. Hayakawa, S. I. In G. Kepes. (1995). *The Language of Vision.* New York: Dover, p. 10.

CHAPTER 8

1. Isaacs, W. (1999). *Dialogue and the Art of Thinking Together: A Pioneering Approach to Communicating in Business and in Life.* New York: Currency.

2. Campbell, J. (1968). *The Hero with a Thousand Faces.* Princeton, NJ: Princeton University Press.

3. Isaacs, W. (1994). Dialogue. In P. Senge, R. Ross, B. Smith, C. Roberts, & A. Kleiner (Eds.), *The Fifth Discipline Fieldbook: Strategies and Tools for Building a Learning Organization.* New York: Currency, pp. 357–364.

4. Habermas, J. (1979). *Communication and the Evolution of Society.* (T. McCarthy, Trans.) Boston: Beacon Press, p. 2.

5. Alexander, C. (1979). *The Timeless Way of Building.* New York: Oxford University Press.

6. Waitzkin, H. (2000). *The Second Sickness: Contradictions of Capitalist Healthcare.* Lanham, MD: Rowman & Littlefield.

7. Covey, S. R. (1989). *The Seven Habits of Highly Effective People: Restoring the Character Ethic.* New York: Simon & Schuster.

8. Moffitt, P. (2002, January/February). Forgiving the unforgivable. *Yoga Journal,* pp. 59–65.

9. Moffitt. Forgiving the unforgivable, pp. 59–65.

10. Jung, C. M., von Franz, M. L., Henderson, J. L., Jacobi, J., & Jaffé, A. (1964). *Man and His Symbols.* Garden City, NY: Doubleday.

11. Whitmont, E. C. (1993). *The Alchemy of Healing: Psyche and Soma.* Berkeley, CA: North Atlantic Books.

12. Ellinor, L., & Gerard, G. (1998). *Dialogue: Rediscover the Transforming Power of Conversation.* New York: John Wiley & Sons, pp. 45–54.

13. Saunders, M. (2001). Personal communication.

CHAPTER 9

1. Barasch, M. I. (1993). *The Healing Path: A Soul Approach to Illness.* New York: Jeremy P. Tarcher, p. 311.

2. Barasch, M. I. (1993). *The Healing Path: A Soul Approach to Illness.* New York: Jeremy P. Tarcher, p. 311.

3. Katz, R., Biesele, M., & St. Denis, V. (1997). *Healing Makes Our Hearts Happy: Spirituality & Cultural Transformation among the Kalahari Ju/'hoansi.* Rochester, VT: Inner Traditions, pp. 141–142.

4. Von Korff, M., Gruman, J., Schaefer, J., & Wagner, E. H. (1997). Collaborative management of chronic illness. *Annals of Internal Medicine, 127,* 1097–1102.

5. Von Korff, ibid.

6. Hudler, J. (July 2001). Personal communication.

7. Cameron, J. (April 2000). Personal communication.

8. Cacchione, P. (February 2001). Personal communication.

9. Glaser, J. (August 2001). Personal communication.

Selected Bibliography

Aaron, H. J., & Schwartz, W. B. (1984). *The Painful Prescription: Rationing Health Care.* Washington, D.C.: Brookings Institute.

Alexander, C. (1979). *The Timeless Way of Building.* New York: Oxford University Press.

Amick, B. C., Levine, S., Tarlov, A. R., & Walsh, D. C. (Eds.). (1995). *Society and Health.* New York: Oxford University Press.

Anspaugh, D. J., Hamrick, M. H., & Rosato, F. D. (1997). *Wellness: Concepts and Applications.* St. Louis, MO: Mosby.

Argyris, Chris. (1986, September). Skilled incompetence. *Harvard Business Review.*

Barasch, M. I. (1993). *The Healing Path: A Soul Approach to Illness.* New York: Jeremy P. Tarcher.

Becker, E. (1973). *The Denial of Death.* New York: Free Press.

Berkman, L. F., & Kawachi, I. (2000). *Social Epidemiology.* New York: Oxford University Press.

Berwick, D. (1990). *Curing Health Care: New Strategies for Quality Improvement: A Report on the National Demonstration Project on Quality Improvement in Health Care.* San Francisco: Jossey-Bass.

Bohm, D., & Edwards, M. (1991). *Changing Consciousness.* New York: Harper San Francisco.

Brandon, R. M., Podhorzer, M., Pollak, T. H. (1992). Premiums without benefits: Waste and inefficiency in the commercial insurance industry. In V. Navarro (Ed.), *Why the United States Does Not Have a National Health Program.* Amityville, NY: Baywood.

Brown, E. R. (1979). *Rockefeller Medicine Men: Medicine and Capitalism in America.* Berkeley: University of California Press.

Byock, Ira. (1997). *Dying Well: The Prospect for Growth at the End of Life.* New York: Riverhead Books.

Callahan, D. (1977). Health and Society: Some Ethical Imperatives. In J.H. Knowles (Ed.), *Doing Better and Feeling Worse: Health in the United States.* New York: Norton.

Campbell, J. (1968). *The Hero with a Thousand Faces.* Princeton, NJ: Princeton University Press.

Caplan, A. L., Engelhardt, H. T., & McCartney, J.J. (Eds.). (1981). *Concepts of Health and Disease: Interdisciplinary Perspectives.* Reading, MA: Addison-Wesley.

Clanham-Clyne, J., Himmelstein, D., & Woodhandler, S. (1995). *The Regional Option for a National Health Program.* Stony Creek, CT: Pamphleteer's Press.

Conrad, P. (Ed.). (1997). *The Sociology of Health and Illness: Critical Perspectives* (5th ed.). New York: St. Martin's Press.

Cousins, N. (1979). *Anatomy of an Illness as Perceived by the Patient: Reflections on Healing and Regeneration.* New York: Norton.

Coverage Matters: Insurance and Health Care. (2001). National Academy Press. Available: http://books.nap.edu/html/coveragematters

Covey, S. R. (1989). *The Seven Habits of Highly Effective People: Restoring the Character Ethic.* New York: Simon & Schuster.

Dembe, A. E. (1996). *Occupation and Disease: How Social Factors Affect the Conception of Work-Related Disorders.* New Haven, CT: Yale University Press.

Deming, E. W. (1986). *Out of the Crisis.* Cambridge, MA: MIT Press.

Durkheim, E. (1951). *Suicide.* New York: Free Press.

Ellinor, L., & Gerard, G. (1998). *Dialogue: Rediscover the Transforming Power of Conversation.* New York: John Wiley & Sons.

Erlich, P. R. & Erlich, A. H. (1991). *Healing the Planet: Strategies for Resolving the Environmental Crisis.* Boston: Addison-Wesley.

Evans, R. G., Barer, M. L., & Marmor, T. R. (Eds.). (1994). *Why Are Some People Healthy and Others Not? The Determinants of Health of Populations.* New York: Aldine De Gruyter.

Feldstein, P.J. (1988). *The Politics of Health Legislation: An Economic Perspective.* Ann Arbor, MI: Health Administration Press.

Findlay, S., & Miller, J. (1999). *Down a Dangerous Path: The Erosion of Health Insurance Coverage.* National Coalition on Health Care. Available: www.nchc.org/releases/erosion.html

Flood, R. L. (1999). *Rethinking the Fifth Discipline: Learning within the Unknowable.* New York: Routledge.

Frank, A. W. (1995). *The Wounded Storyteller: Body, Illness, and Ethics.* Chicago: University of Chicago Press.

Greenberg, W. (1998). *The Health Care Market Place.* New York: Springer.

Gussow, Z. (1989). *Leprosy, Racism, and Public Health: Social Policy in Chronic Disease Control.* Boulder, CO: Westview Press.

Habermas, J. (1979). *Communication and the Evolution of Society.* (T. McCarthy, Trans.) Boston: Beacon Press.

Helms, R. B. (Ed.). (1997). *American Health Policy: Critical Issues for Reform.* Washington, D.C.: DAEI Press.

Hilfiker, D., M.D. (1994). *Not All of Us Are Saints: A Doctor's Journey with the Poor.* New York: Hill & Wang.

Howe, R. L. (1963). *The Miracle of Dialogue.* Greenwich, CT: Seaburg Press.

Institute of Medicine Committee on Quality Health Care in America. (2001). *Crossing the Quality Chasm: A New Health System for the 21st Century*. Washington, D.C.: National Academy Press.

Isaacs, W. (1999). *Dialogue and the Art of Thinking Together: A Pioneering Approach to Communicating in Business and in Life*. New York: Currency.

Jung, C. M., von Franz, M. L., Henderson, J. L., Jacobi, J., & Jaffé, A. (1964). *Man and His Symbols*. Garden City, NY: Doubleday.

Katz, R., Biesele, M., & St. Denis, V. (1997). *Healing Makes Our Hearts Happy: Spirituality & Cultural Transformation among the Kalahari Ju/'hoansi*. Rochester, VT: Inner Traditions.

Kawachi, I., Kennedy, B. P., & Wilkinson, R. G. (Eds.). (1999). *The Society and Population Health Reader: Vol. 1. Income Inequality and Health*. New York: New Press.

Kepes, G. (1995). *The Language of Vision*. New York: Dover.

Lee, P. R., Estes, C. L., & Ramsay, N. (Eds.). (1994). *The Nation's Health* (4th ed.). Boston: Jones and Bartlett.

Mairs, N. (2001). *A Troubled Guest: Life and Death Stories*. Boston: Beacon Press.

Maslow, A. H. (1968). *Toward a Psychology of Being*. New York: Van Nostrand Reinhold.

Maxwell, S., Moon M., & Sega, M. (Dec. 2000). *Growth in Medicare and Out-of-Pocket Spending: Impact on Vulnerable Beneficiaries*. Urban Institute. Available: www.urban.org/health/growth-in-medicare.html

McKeown, T. (1988). *The Origins of Human Disease*. New York: Blackwell.

Meadows, D., Meadows, D., & Randers, J. (1992). *Beyond the Limits: Confronting Global Collapse, Envisioning a Sustainable Future*. Post Mills, VT: Chelsea Green.

Mechanic, D. (1994). *Inescapable Decisions: The Imperatives of Health Reform*. New Brunswick, NJ: Transaction Publishers.

Morreim, E. H. (1995). *Balancing Act: The New Medical Ethics of Medicine's New Economics*. Washington, D.C.: Georgetown University Press.

National Civic League. (1993). *The Healthy Communities Handbook*. Denver: National Civic League.

Navarro, V. (Ed.). (1992). *Why the United States Does Not Have a National Health Program*. Amityville, NY: Baywood.

Ornish, D. (1998). *Love and Survival: The Scientific Basis for the Healing Power of Intimacy*. New York: HarperCollins.

Rawls, J. (1971). *A Theory of Justice*. Cambridge, MA: Belknap Press.

Salmon, J. W. (Ed). (1994). *The Corporate Transformation of Health Care: Perspectives & Implications.*, NY: Baywood.

Senge, P. (1990). *The Fifth Discipline: The Art and Practice of the Learning Organization.* New York: Doubleday.

Senge, P., Ross, R., Smith, B., Roberts, C., & Kleiner, A. (Eds.) (1994). *The Fifth Discipline Fieldbook: Strategies and Tools for Building a Learning Organization*. New York: Currency.

Sontag, S. (1978). *Illness as Metaphor*. New York: Farrar, Straus & Giroux.

Starr, P. (1982). *The Social Transformation of American Medicine*. New York: Basic Books.

Starr, P. (1994). *The Logic of Health-Care Reform*. New York: Whittle Books.

Stein, H. F. (1990). *American Medicine as Culture.* Boulder, CO: Westview Press.

Stewart, C. T. (1995). *Healthy, Wealthy or Wise: Issues in American Health Care Policy.* Armonk, NY: M.E. Sharpe.

Strosberg, M A., Wiener, J. M., Baker, R., & Fein, I. A. (1992). *Rationing America's Medical Care: The Oregon Plan and Beyond.* Washington, D.C.: Brookings Institute.

Tarlov, A. R., & St. Peter, R. F. (Eds.) (2000). *The Society and Population Health Reader: A State and Community Perspective.* New York: New Press.

Taylor, F. W. (1967). *The Principles of Scientific Management.* New York: Norton.

United Nations International Covenant on Economic, Social, and Cultural Rights (1967). Available: http://www.unchr.html/menu3/b/a_cescr.htm

Waitzkin, H. (1983). *The Second Sickness: Contradictions of Capitalist Health Care.* New York: Free Press.

Waitzkin, H. (2000). *The Second Sickness: Contradictions of Capitalist Health Care.* Lanham, MD: Rowman & Littlefield.

Whitmont, E. C. (1993). *The Alchemy of Healing: Psyche and Soma.* Berkeley, CA: North Atlantic Books.

Wilber, K. (1995). *Sex, Ecology, Spirituality: The Spirit of Evolution.* Boston: Shambhala.

Index

About the Author

BARBARA J. SOWADA is a fellow in the Healthcare Forum's Healthier Communities Fellowship.